THE
STOLEN
YEAR

THE
STOLEN
YEAR

How COVID Changed Children's Lives,
and Where We Go Now

ANYA KAMENETZ

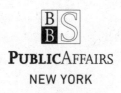

PUBLICAFFAIRS

NEW YORK

PublicAffairs
Hachette Book Group
1290 Avenue of the Americas, New York, NY 10104
www.publicaffairsbooks.com
@Public_Affairs

Printed in the United States of America

First Edition: August 2022

Published by PublicAffairs, an imprint of Perseus Books, LLC, a subsidiary of Hachette Book Group, Inc. The PublicAffairs name and logo is a trademark of the Hachette Book Group.

The Hachette Speakers Bureau provides a wide range of authors for speaking events. To find out more, go to www.hachettespeakersbureau.com or call (866) 376-6591.

The publisher is not responsible for websites (or their content) that are not owned by the publisher.

Print book interior design by Trish Wilkinson

Library of Congress Cataloging-in-Publication Data
Names: Kamenetz, Anya, 1980– author.
Title: The stolen year : how COVID changed children's lives, and where we go now / Anya Kamenetz.
Description: First edition. | New York : PublicAffairs, [2022]
Identifiers: LCCN 2022001106 | ISBN 9781541700987 (hardcover) | ISBN 9781541701014 (ebook)
Subjects: LCSH: Education—Social aspects—United States—History—21st century. | COVID-19 Pandemic, 2020—Social aspects—United States. | Children—United States—Social conditions—21st century. | Child welfare—United States—History—21st century. | Educational sociology—United States.
Classification: LCC LC191.4 .K36 2022 | DDC 306.430973/0905—dc23/eng/20220524
LC record available at https://lccn.loc.gov/2022001106

ISBNs: 9781541700987 (hardcover), 9781541701014 (ebook)

LSC-C

Printing 1, 2022

A Note

Where people are identified by first names only, those names and sometimes other minor details have been changed to protect their privacy—with the exception of David, in Chapter 6, who I originally interviewed for NPR and agreed to use his real first name only. Heather, in St. Louis, chose the pseudonyms for herself and her children.

Contents

INTRODUCTION

In early March 2020, Dr. Dara Kass sat down with her three children at home in Park Slope, Brooklyn, and told them they were going to stay with her parents in New Jersey for a while. "Think of it like summer camp," she said.

"Am I going to die?" seven-year-old Sammy asked.

A slender goofball who likes to sneak into his dad's study to use his VR headset, Sammy had a liver transplant when he was two years old to reverse the progress of a rare genetic disorder. Dara was the donor. He still has a compromised immune system, still takes meds daily. It's not so unusual for him to ask whether something could kill him. "Sammy talks about his mortality—not all the time, but he does understand that his life is, in some way, precious," his mother says.

Dara had started to see her emergency room fill up with patients with cough, fever, and shortness of breath. She'd also seen the preliminary data from China, showing how easily the novel coronavirus spread within households.

Dark-haired, short, and straight to the point, Dara chose other people's worst-case scenarios to be her everyday routine. She doesn't find it "helpful" to dwell on feelings. She's a problem solver. She has the knowledge and research skills to fuel endless cycles of anxiety and planning, so she tries to avoid spiraling. "My rabbit holes are deep," she says. "But they're not frequent, because I go places people don't even know."

But with a looming global pandemic, she had no choice. "I started figuring out—I started playing a game in my mind. How do you quarantine your family from you if you're positive or even exposed? And I started thinking about the floors of my house and the rooms and the bathrooms—and most specifically I want to protect my youngest."

Dara decided the safest course of action was to quarantine her children with her parents in New Jersey for a few weeks while she continued to work at the hospital. "I put them all together in the same house and said, OK, figure it out and I'm going to worry about work."

She dropped off Sammy, ten-year-old Charlie, and twelve-year-old Hannah on Friday, March 13, and hugged them tight. Hannah put on a brave face, but she was worried. Dara couldn't say when she'd see them again.

Dara worked twenty-four hours at an increasingly hectic hospital over the weekend. Monday morning she woke up feeling like she'd been stabbed in the back. Her coffee tasted like hot water.

Across the country in San Francisco, eleven-year-old Jonah and his mother, Maya, walked out of a parent-teacher conference on March 12 that had actually gone well. After two years of phone calls, meetings, lobbying, paperwork, fights, and frustration, he was getting support for his dyslexia in small groups at school. His English scores were up two hundred points in the past few months. A behavioral therapist was coming to the house almost every day to help reinforce desired behaviors like sitting at dinner and taking conversational turns. His team was discussing Jonah "graduating" from his behavioral therapy. A handsome boy with a round face and a mop of brown curls, Jonah spoke up for himself in the meeting and was proud of his progress. Things were getting better at home too. Jonah's moods were steadier. He was less likely to explode at Maya's fiancé, Robert, or at Robert's teenage son, Rust.

Robert works in health education. Lately he had been tasked with designing teaching materials about this novel virus. "Basically, I spent a good part of a week with my colleagues making slide decks for students about washing your hands, staying away from people, social distancing."

Maya got an alert on her phone as she walked out of the parent-teacher conference: San Francisco public schools announced a three-week closure. It was an "oh shit" moment.

"I'm scared," Jonah told his mother at bedtime that night, in his upstairs room with a view that peeks at the Bay. He was afraid his progress would disappear without the support he was used to. That without the routine of school, recess, and friends, he would start acting, in his words, "crazy."

Two days later in rural Oklahoma, on Saturday, March 14, Jeannie teared up in line at the Aldi's grocery. The guy in front of her looked like he was hoarding. "We call them corn-fed here, like a big farmer guy. He had a cartful of chicken and potatoes. And I thought, I really hope you're buying that for your elderly grandparents or something because you don't need to be buying all that out from under everybody else." Her cart was full, too, but then again she had five kids at home.

Beneath her resentment, Jeannie remembers a spooky, sinking feeling. "I just felt like, this was not the world I'm supposed to be in. Like, never in my life would I ever've thought that this would be my life."

In the Deanwood neighborhood of Washington, DC, a baby boy named Patrick was cranky without his usual routine at daycare and showing physical discomfort. He was born with a genetic disorder called Noonan syndrome, which can cause heart defects, other physical abnormalities, and developmental delays. His physical and speech therapy sessions were all canceled. His older brother, Pete Jr., had cabin fever, running around the house pretending to be Batman.

Their dad, Pete, had to head back out to work at the end of March, after just two weeks at home. His job as a groundskeeper on a golf course had been deemed "essential" by the city. Their mother Patricia's job as an aide in a special education class was on pause as the district figured out its distance learning plan. Patricia was "in disbelief."

"My biggest fear as a little girl getting married was always being in the house, having to always clean it. And then I was like, I don't want to be, like, *The Help*, either." For a professional Black woman with a master's degree, being stuck in the house all day with two little boys felt like being sent back in time. "I would never have been a good house slave. I would have been killed. Right? I know they would have killed me. I felt like I was drowning."

This is a book about Sammy's fear of dying and Patricia's feeling of drowning. Jonah's support network evaporating. Jeannie's spooky, sinking feeling.

About the experiences of children and the people who loved them during the first year of the pandemic.

Since 2014, I've covered education as a correspondent for National Public Radio. I used to have this mini–pep talk I would give about why education was a worthy beat for a journalist. I would say, This country doesn't have universal health care. We are profoundly weak at providing subsidized affordable housing, mass transit, or other public goods. We have no childcare system to speak of. No paid family leave. But we do have this beautiful phenomenon where in every neighborhood, in every city, town, and rural community in America, there is a warm, lighted building that children can go to for 180 days a year. There they will be safe, they will be fed, and they are likely to encounter a caring adult or two and maybe even learn something. All for free.

Yes, our schools are segregated, inequitable, and starved for resources. They fail too many. But they have kept the lights on year after year for fifty million children. And in 2020 this was all taken away, with no adequate substitute. Our society did not muster the resources or the will to take care of our children anymore, to offer these basics.

As March 2020 turned to April and then May, it dawned on all of us that, in so many ways, the cavalry wasn't coming. Institutions and leaders weren't taking the necessary steps to make sure children's needs were met, for food, care, education, or connection.

Hundreds of children ultimately died directly of COVID-19. This is a tragedy. We were fortunate that this direct toll was not larger. Instead, the harm of the pandemic for the overwhelming majority of children came in a host of other forms.

A full year into the pandemic, more than four in ten children were still not attending school in person. That was not the norm in most parts of other wealthy countries, regardless of the many different courses of their pandemics.

The federal school lunch program, the second-largest public food program, was reduced to handing out paper bags with sandwiches in parking lots. Child hunger skyrocketed. In April 2020, 17.5 percent of parents told the Census Bureau that their young children actually weren't getting enough to eat—something that is usually too rare to appear in the data. "It's just unthinkable," scholar Diane Schanzenbach told me. "These are just levels that we've never seen before."

Parents lucky enough to have paid jobs had to choose every day between working, sleeping, and taking care of their children and often failed at all three. Mothers were forced out of the workforce by the millions, which will ultimately drive more children into poverty. Domestic workers, nannies, and the other invisible hands who care for children day in and day out were left without income, had little access to government aid, and were driven from the field.

Children missed basic medical care like vaccinations. Depression, anxiety, suicidality, obesity, eating disorders, and diabetes climbed. Nearly two hundred thousand US children were bereaved and orphaned as the uncontrolled pandemic raged on.

Children's pain seems to command extra attention. But too often people want to wish it away. And so I want to be clear: some, likely even most, of our kids will put this year behind them. But they all had something taken from them.

I've been thinking of this book as a little like restorative justice or therapy. It tells the story of 2020 and 2021 in the words of children and teenagers from around the country, especially those who are often overlooked.

This was a time of quarantine, an economy that crumpled like a paper cup, limited in-person school and childcare, fear, anxiety, grief, soul-crushing monotony, traumatic levels of stress, and isolation.

Plus white supremacist terrorist violence, historic antiracist protests, a failed coup and insurrection, rampant anti-science misinformation and disinformation pushed at the highest levels of government. New records in natural disasters, from fires to hurricanes to ice storms. The death of more than half a million Americans from a new virus in a single year (a number that just keeps growing).

It also was a year that many children were able to spend at home with their families. Researchers affirmed that there was a buffer for these children and their caregivers in simply being together.

We, the people who hopelessly love children, filtered 2020 for them as much as we could. Like a mask, we laid down multiple protective layers of love, playfulness, and electronic distraction.

We camped in the backyard, built pillow forts, taught our kids to read, supported them when they struggled. They saw us struggling, too, barking at each other, crying when it all got to be too much. We sang and danced and read stories over Zoom. We returned to the exhaustion we'd known as parents of newborns, discovered new reserves of energy we didn't know we had, and then burned those up, too, as we wondered when this would ever end.

And against all odds, as they always do, our children grew.

I reported and wrote this book largely from my six-by-eight-foot home office in Brooklyn with one or both of my daughters elsewhere in the house. My husband and I had part-time childcare from the beginning thanks to our downstairs neighbor.

I talked to the families mentioned in this book over Zoom and by phone in the thick of things; we didn't meet in person until after vaccination.

This book is a testimony of fierce love. Family members, caregivers, teachers, social workers, pediatricians, therapists, bus drivers, classroom aides, food service staff, and crossing guards stretched beyond their limits to protect children throughout this year. Individuals did as much as they could.

But it wasn't enough.

"This could affect a whole generation for the rest of their lives," Dr. Jack Shonkoff, a pediatrician and director of the Center on the Developing Child at Harvard University, told a reporter in July 2021. "All kids will be affected. Some will get through this and be fine. They will learn from it and grow. But lots of kids are going to be in big trouble."

Dara's children were among the luckiest. After she recovered from COVID, they spent most of the pandemic in a three-story brownstone in Park Slope with both parents and an au pair from Mexico. Dara and her husband, Michael, a hedge-fund manager, remodeled their basement into a one-room schoolhouse and hired a "pod" teacher. Sammy was able to do third grade in safe company and see friends in person every day. He also loved seeing way more of his parents than usual.

Their middle child, Charlie, never much cared for school anyway. He liked getting up early, having a bowl of Cinnamon Toast Crunch in peace, speeding through his work, and having plenty of time to dedicate to YouTube. "Mommy, it's a pandemic, but I'm kind of living my best life," he told Dara. "Everyone around me is anxious. I'm doing just fine. I like this life, you know? I'm eleven years old. Everything is given to me. I don't have to leave my house."

Hannah, their oldest, was by turns despondent and enraged, but not necessarily out of the bounds of normal puberty. She watched all seventeen seasons of the hospital melodrama *Grey's Anatomy* in the first couple of months, as her mother was going to work at the actual hospital. Her blowout bat mitzvah was scaled down to a small gathering. "I'm really bored," she told me. "The isolation aspect is really hard. I think that we lost a lot of hope for things."

Children like these, the luckiest kids in the country, had to confront death in a way that most privileged children in the United States have not had to for decades.

My own two girls are among them. They lost school, time with their friends, milestones. A year of development, learning, experience was altered beyond recognition. They will be telling this story for the rest of their lives, and it will shape their futures. This book is about them.

Other kids weren't so lucky. The effects of this year will not be so subtle. And they can't be waved away with happy talk about "resilience." Their parents lost work, stood in line for food. Their homes, which they could not leave, were unsafe. They, or their parents, or both, developed serious mental health problems. They regressed without therapies and interventions. There was no one to make sure they went to school on the computer, or online learning just wasn't doable for them and they disconnected. Their neighborhoods got more violent and more divided. They were quarantined alone. They weren't allowed to see their families in person for up to a year. This is their story too.

In March 2021, the *New York Times* asked a group of pediatric infectious disease specialists about the impact on children of this first year of COVID. Their answers formed a litany of woe. "Food insecurity. Socialization. Depression. Isolation.... Children are suffering academically, emotionally, socially and physically.... The long-term consequences may not be fully realized for years.... We are going to have a lost generation—a set of children who will fall behind educationally, with deficits that could affect their entire life course."

Sound points. Echoed by the experts you will hear from throughout this book. Yet this article ran a calendar year into the pandemic! For most of that time, and since, our country has continued failing to put children at the center of our decision making to prevent or remedy these eventualities, even though they were foreseen from the very beginning.

We did grave harm to children simply by failing to consider their needs at all.

A second category of harm, less infuriating but maybe more confounding, was done out of misplaced care. This disease was novel and unusual. It tricked our intuition and experience by being much, much less of a threat to children than it was to adults. And so, particularly in the most progressive parts of the country, adults prolonged school closures and other restrictions.

We ended up with closed playgrounds next to open dog parks, closed schools next door to open bars, and eventually a nearly opened-up country with no vaccines for children.

All of this was not inevitable. In the words of feminist author and activist Eve Rodsky, it was "super fucking *evitable.*"

The crisis exposed fault lines that run to the core. Why are our schools left to feed thirty million hungry children? Why does a single public school building in the United States of America lack soap, paper towels, or running water in the bathrooms? Why are one in thirty children homeless? Why do we not provide a public subsidy so that the people who help take care of our children can make a living wage? Why no paid family leave? Why is it such a battle to get legally mandated services for children in special education? Why do children wait years to get mental health care? Why are such heavy government apparatuses set up to incarcerate children and separate them from their families—especially Black, Brown, and immigrant children— and relative scraps dedicated to help those families stay intact?

These are the kinds of questions that require a dive into history. Each chapter will give you some of that background.

I witnessed the aftermath of Hurricane Katrina as a young journalist. What was true then is true of all disasters. When collapses like this happen, fault lines become obvious to everyone. And when we rebuild, there is a chance to remake.

The pandemic isn't over.

The story of what happened to children during the pandemic isn't over by a long shot.

The decisions that led us here were made by powerful adults over centuries. The adults of today are at the start of what must be a generation-long process of redressing harms done to children. This is not the last global crisis they are going to see in their lives—this is a perilous world indeed we have brought them into. Our responses now will be decisive going forward.

This story is not over in another way. It's ultimately up to our children to define their own experiences of what happened this year and why. Not one of them is doomed. And we owe it to them to listen. This book is one attempt at that.

1   SCHOOLS

We're prepared, and we're doing a great job with it. And it will go away. Just stay calm. It will go away.

—President Trump, March 10, 2020

March 10, 2020, US seven-day average of cases: 128

IN OKLAHOMA

A nine-year-old girl named Ruby is standing on a balance beam. Her rope of black hair hangs past her waist. She is crying very quietly. Advanced in skills, she is the tiniest girl in the class. The markers on the beam, showing where she needs to jump for this drill, have been placed too wide for her. At this moment she is afraid of the leap to come.

This is the last gymnastics class before lockdown.

Ruby is growing up in a little white farmhouse on a state highway close to the Cherokee Nation. She lives with her mother, two teenage brothers, and two younger sisters, twins. Her parents are divorced, but her dad still lives in the house too.

Everyone calls her sisters "the babies" and treats them that way, though they are only two years younger than Ruby. The girls' room is dim, stacked with bunk beds. It reeks from the live crickets Ruby feeds to her three frogs, Janis Hoplin, Green Simmons, and John Froggerty. She likes the frogs' big eyes, their friendly-looking faces.

The beginning of the pandemic was "weird, like a movie." They went on spring break and just…never came back. Ruby didn't really understand what started it. She didn't know why different people she knew believed different things about it, and why some people didn't want to wear a mask if that was supposed to keep you safe.

She turned ten in March 2020. No party. Her mom got two different cheesecakes, her favorite, from two different grocery stores, and they watched *Jumanji*. Her big brothers, Julian and Rob, didn't bother to wish her a happy birthday. "They hardly come out of their rooms."

"I ALWAYS HAD SCHOOL"

Ruby's mom, Jeannie, is a teacher at the only school in town. Just a few miles down the road from the little white farmhouse is a ramble of run-down buildings dating from the 1930s through the 1990s. Many of Jeannie's students didn't have computers or internet at home. So when school closed, Jeannie and some colleagues went into the empty main building, which she swears is haunted, to make up paper assignments and use the copy machine. "We kind of just handed out packets and said, you know, good luck."

The state of Oklahoma ranks forty-eighth in spending per student in its public schools. Jeannie teaches sixth-grade English in a town of less than two thousand people, earning $48,000 a year. She can't imagine doing anything else. "One reason I went into teaching is for the job stability, because there's always going to be teachers," she says. "My school has been my stable point because it's always there."

Jeannie doesn't just teach here—she also went here, as have her children. "I'm forty-one and I want to say, like, thirty-five years of my life have been here. Through my whole life that's where I went—to school. When my home life was in turmoil, I always had school."

When Jeannie was four years old, her mom divorced her dad. Her mother was a beauty, petite and dark like Ruby. She soon remarried. "It was back and forth, back and forth. In the summer we would move out and then she'd go back to my stepdad. She had my brother when I was ten or eleven." Jeannie was raised a lot by her grandmother.

One time Jeannie was driving with her daughters, and they spotted her mother walking by the roadside. "Look, babies," Ruby said to her little sisters. "That's Grandma." The twins pressed their faces to the window of the van to catch a glimpse.

Jeannie and her children are registered members of the Cherokee Nation in Oklahoma, one of nearly six hundred federally recognized Indigenous tribes in the United States. That means they can trace their ancestry back to the Dawes Rolls, a federal census of the Cherokees, Creeks, Choctaws, Chickasaws, and Seminoles taken around the turn of the twentieth century. She and her family are among the seven in ten Native Americans who live off reservations.

Jeannie is one-thirty-second Cherokee on her mother's side, and the rest white. Her ex, George, is more or less the reverse—mostly Cherokee and Cree, just one-thirty-second white. Native identity is complex, and official tribal membership is not the same thing as community acceptance. She and her kids never felt welcome at her in-laws. "All of his brothers and sisters married Native Americans. And so if I were to go over there on holidays and things like that, I would be the only white person over there. And, like, understandably so, they don't like white people."

For Ruby, the concept of grandparents is so foggy that when she was little, she got the words "grandpa" and "grandma" mixed up. George's parents are teachers of the Cherokee language, but his kids aren't sure whether they feel Native.

So it's been the school, more than family, that has anchored them to a town whose main street is a row of vacant storefronts.

Jeannie daydreams about moving away. "I think the main reason I haven't is because I can't let go of something that's been my stability all my life. I mean, it's just always been there."

SCHOOLS CLOSE AROUND THE WORLD

Always, until 2020. Within a ten-day period in mid-March, schools in all fifty states, the District of Columbia, and Puerto Rico shut their doors. So did schools around the world, affecting 1.4 billion children at the peak.

When schools closed, the virus was still little more than a rumor across much of this country. At the time people spoke in terms of a two- or three-week extended spring break. But only a few hundred of the nation's fifty-six million K–12 students would see the inside of a school building again that academic year. As of January 2021, a year from the official start of the pandemic, more than half the world's student population still faced disrupted learning. More than four in ten US students were still in remote school, including a majority of children of color.

Schools closed in some of the US for the influenza pandemic in 1917–1918 and for polio outbreaks in the 1940s. For SARS in Beijing in 2003; for swine flu in Mexico City, some Texas districts, New York City, and elsewhere in the United States in 2009; and regularly, seasonally, through the 2010s for the flu in countries including Russia and Japan. In addition to keeping children from contact with each other in classrooms, closing schools is intended to reduce crowding on public transit and to keep parents home to watch their children. These more recent closures were much shorter and more limited than what happened in the United States during COVID.

While always recognized as costly, school closures weren't as widespread or disruptive in earlier decades as they were likely to be in 2020. In 1918 and in the 1940s, enrollment overall was much lower. High school graduation rates didn't cross 50 percent in this country until the end of the Second World War. Fewer women were working and thus reliant on school for childcare.

Since the mid-twentieth century, closing schools nationwide for months on end has happened only during major social breakdowns, like those brought on by a refugee crisis, a war, or a natural disaster. One of the world's experts on this topic is Rebecca Winthrop, a senior fellow at the Brookings Institution, who helped popularize "education in emergencies"—the concept that education should be an integral and swift part of international disaster response.

"There is a lot of literature on the impact of crises on children," she told me in March 2020. "And it's particularly on children's psychosocial well-being that school closures, that disruption in routine, [have] the largest effect."

DISCONNECTED YOUTH AFTER KATRINA

I had eyewitness experience of this. New Orleans is my hometown. In the fall of 2005 and the spring of 2006 I reported on the aftermath of Hurricane Katrina. The storm shuttered public schools in the city for several months.

I keep a photo on my computer desktop. I took it outside the River Center, a stadium turned storm shelter in Baton Rouge, Louisiana, on a hot weekday afternoon in September 2005. Three Black boys pose in crisp white undershirts that defy the humidity and the squalor of shelter life. J., the youngest, looks at the camera, arms slung over the shoulders of his cousins. M. has his hands clasped in front of him, fingertips steepled, and gazes pensively off to the side. His older brother S. is looking down.

They told me they had waited out the storm at a Days Inn and were bussed from the New Orleans Superdome to Arkansas, where they attended a few days of school and were bullied for being "storm kids." Then, for some reason, they were taken back to Louisiana, where I found them tossing a football around.

When I asked them why they were not in school that day, S. shook his head. "I don't want to. I just don't want to go. Just don't." His cousin piped up, "You're scared of the kids there!"

Many of Katrina's children, like these boys, scattered across the map. They went to Baton Rouge, Houston, even Salt Lake City. Doug Harris, at Tulane University, tracked the ones who eventually came back.

Some had been out of classes for only a few weeks. They had almost immediately enrolled in school, usually a better-funded, higher-performing school, elsewhere. Nevertheless, it took them more than two years, until the spring of 2008, to catch up to where they had been academically.

"The disruption and everything that went along with Katrina did hamper them. The lost school time, anxiety, the economic insecurity, all those factors together—it's hard to isolate the school effect." Teenagers fared worst. They ran out of time to catch up. They were more likely to have other concerns, like the need to work to support a family.

The collective trauma of the "storm kids" lingered into the next generation. Ten years after the storm, in 2015, New Orleans had one of the highest percentages of "disconnected youth" of any city in the country: almost one in five were neither working nor in school. And even by 2020, fifteen years later, Harris told me, enrollment in New Orleans public and community colleges was still below what it had been. A boy with the same name and age as one of those I met outside the River Center was arrested for homicide there in 2013, at the age of twenty-two.

In the fall of 2021, Hurricane Ida once again closed schools for about 150,000 children for a few weeks in New Orleans and for even longer in the harder-hit outlying parishes. The storm strengthened over the climate-heated gulf with unforeseen speed. Students and teachers went home for the weekend without bringing laptops and hotspots, even if they had them. And then there were the power outages, stretching for up to a month in some areas. Harris told me that the displacement, and the impact of Ida on those children, were likely to last even longer than that of Katrina. We are living in an era where human-induced disasters rain fresh blows on already-bruised skin. We need to get a lot better at education in emergencies.

TWO THINGS CHILDREN AND FAMILIES NEED

"There is a big social shift you have to think about when schools stay closed for long periods of time," Winthrop told me when we spoke at the very beginning of the crisis. "Amazingly, kids are pretty resilient. But you have to find ways to give them two things." First:

> a normal sense of routine. It doesn't have to be the exact replica of schooling, but if you give them a normal sense of routine with enough activities throughout the day, it really helps reduce their anxiety and supports their overall psychosocial well-being.
>
> The other thing you need to do is really find deep ways of supporting kids' caregivers, their parents and their teachers. Often people forget until halfway through the emergency response that parents and teachers are also affected by the crisis and they're dealing with their own multitude of problems.

During COVID, the United States didn't do either.

SCHOOL CLOSURE IMPACTS WILL LINGER FOR YEARS

I published a piece on NPR.org on April 2, 2020, outlining measurable consequences that were likely to last for years if schools stayed closed for COVID for even several weeks. It was based on research from New Orleans after Hurricane Katrina, Puerto Rico after Hurricane Maria, and countries across the world: Afghanistan, Argentina, Myanmar, Pakistan, the Philippines, Rwanda, Somalia, Sri Lanka, Syria, Uganda, and Venezuela.

To sum up: When schools close, children don't learn as much math or reading. They may forget what they have already learned. It takes years on average to get back on track. Dropout rates rise. Children are at higher risk of abuse from a parent who is depressed or unemployed, or of an accident when playing unsupervised. They miss hot meals, immunizations, and eye exams. They are vulnerable to early marriage or sex work. They may find themselves having to support their families or care for younger siblings.

This is not to say that every day home from school causes measurable damage to every child. The impact of school closures is wildly unequal. For example, four years after a 2005 earthquake in Pakistan that closed schools for around fourteen weeks, students were on average one and a half years academically behind peers in unaffected regions. Yet children whose mothers had completed primary school, putting them at the top of the local socioeconomic ladder, were unscathed.

A DIFFERENT KIND OF DISASTER

The pandemic has been different from a war, refugee crisis, or natural disaster in at least one important way: families didn't have to flee their homes. Instead, roughly half of workers who were able to work remotely and other caregivers who were out of the workforce, by choice or not, were able to spend more time with their families than ever before. This was an enormous source of solace for many. Love and the daily routines of care buffered us in a terrifying time.

EMERGENCY REMOTE LEARNING: PANIC-GOGY

And of course, the United States did provide a form of education in this emergency. Like the rest of the suddenly remote workforce, teachers had to change everything about how they did their jobs within a matter of days, while being just as sad and scared as everyone else. Teachers around the world made great efforts in a short time to move to "emergency remote learning," "disaster distance learning," or what some instructors dubbed "panic-gogy."

Zoom, the chosen video platform of ninety thousand schools in twenty countries, went from hosting ten million people daily in December 2019 to two hundred million in March 2020.

In these very early days, teachers basked in public approval from parents like the television producer Shonda Rhimes, whose tweet on March 16, 2020, went viral: "Been homeschooling a 6-year old and 8-year old for one hour and 11 minutes. Teachers deserve to make a billion dollars a year. Or a week."

These efforts were big. But just as the research predicted, they fell short. At Jeannie's school, as with schools around the country, there were essentially no more grades given out after March. Grades are not identical with learning. But to her the abandonment of grading was a tacit admission that the social contract of school was broken. "Their parents were supposed to sign saying their children had completed the work. They didn't return it or anything. And that was it. Basically our grades stopped in March. We didn't hold it against the kids who never did anything. So, I mean, really, here their education stopped in March."

RAND, an independent research organization, surveys thousands of teachers regularly. In the spring of 2020, it found 88 percent of teachers said they hadn't covered as much material as they usually would have for the semester, and only one-third were giving out letter grades.

The intention was to avoid penalizing students for circumstances beyond their control. But I also talked to students who complained that loosening requirements sapped their motivation. Like Ricardo, fifteen, who was growing up in foster care in Washington State. "If you're a student like me that has high grades," and they take away the grading part, "you tend to not really care about school at all. I notice at school, sadly, it's not much about learning. It's about getting that grade, about getting that A. And if you only have that grind and the grind stops, it's no more point."

When we talked, Ricardo's face was flipped upside down; there was something going on with his laptop camera. He had been in quarantine for "three weeks and seven days, to be exact" and was getting through his schoolwork in about two hours a day. Then he'd work out, boxing in the garage.

He said he felt lucky to be in a foster placement with his little brother. "Not many kids get that." They were opposites, he said—his brother's passion was basketball. He tried to keep him from focusing too much on the "basketball grind," and his brother helped him loosen up when he was sweating a test.

Ricardo was meeting over Zoom twice a week with his mentor, Dani, from an organization called Treehouse, which has helped raise the high school graduation rate for foster kids in Seattle significantly. "She's been helping me emotionally. It's wonderful what she's been doing." Dani helped provide a structure where school could not. She set up an incentive plan where he could earn Amazon gift cards for "self-care" activities, like doing a puzzle.

A lot of the kids and families I talked to described the same moment as Ricardo—the sound of the gears shifting and the grind coming to a halt.

Jeannie said she heard from maybe half of the parents in her class for the rest of that school year. And her own children didn't fare much better. Ruby mostly did her work without being asked. The boys, thirteen and sixteen, mostly didn't. And Jeannie quickly gave up pushing the "babies," twins April and June. "With my first graders, we did the first few weeks. And that's kind of when it got to the point where I wasn't handling the whole instability of the world very well. And I said, no, this is too much."

CHILDREN ARE DIFFERENT, EVEN SIBLINGS

Jeannie's "babies" were coddled by everyone and never lacked for playmates.

Ruby took over the management of the household. She was alert to, and burdened by, her mother's state of mind. "She sometimes yells. She cries a little bit. I can tell she's stressed out. She's very tired, more than last year. She takes deep breaths and her eyes have bags under them and her glasses, I don't know, they're, like, crooked?"

Jeannie wears scratched-up readers from the grocery store, with red or purple frames. She probably needs a prescription but hasn't bothered to get one.

Rob, a budding metalhead with long hair and black nail polish, had some very dark moments.

Julian, the oldest, is smart and talented. As the research would predict, he was drawn toward paid work and away from academics.

ONLINE LEARNING IS REALLY HARD

Emergency remote learning has been around about as long as broadcast media. During the Second World War, the BBC's existing School Radio program gained a new importance. Any regional variations were consolidated into a single home instructional service for children, with a five-minute news broadcast that was designed to explain the confusing circumstances. By 1942, half of all British schools were listening.

Teachers created an educational radio broadcast in Sierra Leone during the Ebola outbreak in 2014. And just before the pandemic, Sesame Street was developing programming specifically for children in refugee camps in Syria and Bangladesh.

These efforts are considered worthwhile not because they make up for the loss of in-person instruction. They do not. Teachers and aid workers offer them in the faith that they can buffer the stress of the situation and maintain relationships, routines, and hope for children.

However, it's a painful irony that these stopgap efforts themselves multiply inequities. A computer or even a television; a quiet space to work; a grownup literate, confident, and with time and energy to support learning—all of these are privileges.

At the outset of the pandemic, an estimated 15 percent of households with children in the United States lacked high-speed internet. In Ward 7 of Washington, DC, the figure was much higher, 55 percent.

That's where Patricia Stamper lived with her husband, Pete, and their two little boys. Patricia, working at a school, knew how to get her own son a tablet with Wi-Fi, but it took time to get her class set up.

Paper packets were a common fallback plan, and not only in rural areas like Jeannie's. Los Angeles Unified School District teamed with

PBS to broadcast educational TV shows paired with lesson prompts statewide. It was an admission that the second-largest school district in the country was not certain it could reach every child with personal, live online instruction. In the spring of 2020, United Teachers of Los Angeles, the city's teacher union, agreed to just a twenty-hour workweek for remote teaching. The district reported that on an average day that spring, only about 36 percent of middle and high school students participated in online learning. Rates were even lower for Latinx and Black students, those experiencing homelessness, those in the foster care system, and English language learners.

By one estimate, at least three million students around the country didn't meaningfully engage with their education from March to September 2020. As in LA, most of those missing were already on the margin: English language learners, students experiencing housing instability, those with learning disabilities, and migrants. Well into the second pandemic school year, in November 2020, tens of thousands of teachers surveyed reported, on average, being in *contact* with only four out of five students on their class rolls.

The problem with remote school is more than equipment. Prior to the pandemic, very few people thought it was a good idea for students younger than high school age to go to school online.

"Online learning is really hard for a lot of people," says Justin Reich, director of MIT's Teaching Systems Lab. When we talked on March 16, 2020, he called online learning a "force multiplier for inequality."

> People do worse in online learning settings. They get lower grades. They're more likely to drop out and fail. And that "online penalty" is worse for the most vulnerable struggling students in our system.... All of the students who we're most worried about in the pandemic, the students whose parents are most likely to lose their jobs, to be gig workers who are negatively affected, to have inadequate access to health care. Those are all the students that we would predict in advance would struggle most in the transition to online learning.

In San Francisco, eleven-year-old Jonah, who has autism and dyslexia, had finally found a groove in the classroom. This after years of struggling to get a proper special education plan. When school shut down, he had a Chromebook and high-speed internet. San Francisco schools offered live video teaching. But Jonah lost all interest in reading or writing. He was angry and frustrated most of the day. "He's really obsessed with electronics. And so to put him on electronics for school is horrible. He's one of those kids where they're sucked into YouTube," said his stepfather, Robert. He was missing his friends, school, and playing outside.

THE DISASTER ON TOP OF THE DISASTER

Free, universal, high-quality public schools increase social mobility, create a space for individual self-determination, and build economic power in communities. That's the whole point. That's why marginalized groups fight for access to better schools. That's why increasing participation in formal education is a major global development goal. Schools aren't perfect, but on balance they do good.

The converse is also true. Closing school buildings en masse increases inequality and destroys individual hopes and dreams. And the impact can be measured for a generation. That is the disaster on top of the disaster.

BACK TO THE BEGINNING

March 13. It was the vertiginous beginning. The stock market crashed, the NBA canceled its season, Tom Hanks and his wife were diagnosed with coronavirus in Australia.

When Dara, the ER doctor in New York City, was at the nation's epicenter in mid-March, she got a COVID test and it came back positive. Telling her three kids, who were staying with her parents in New Jersey, was the hardest part. She didn't want them to be afraid. She missed them so much already. She tried to joke, over FaceTime, "Don't I make COVID look good?"

"She's definitely really good with, like, sickness and stuff," remembers her oldest, Hannah, who was twelve at the time. "And she's a strong person. But it was kind of scary because I wasn't seeing her. So I couldn't actually see how she was doing. And I had to only see her over the phone. And it was kind of hard."

While she was recuperating, New York was rocketing up the first slope of a surge that peaked on April 4 and would ultimately kill around twenty-three thousand people. "I have [doctor] friends on the phone crying and crying every night. 'It's crazy. People are suffocating in the hallway. We don't have resources.' And it wasn't just one hospital in New York. It was *every* hospital in New York. Brookdale. Elmhurst. This was when we started seeing the refrigerator trucks." Parked outside the hospitals. Makeshift morgues.

Then Dara was out of quarantine, and it was time to get back into the trenches. "I had been imagining what it was like in the ER without seeing it myself. And then I came back from being quarantined and the hospital was full, full, full, and I was kind of emotionally impaired, because I learned over the two weeks that I was home that people were getting sick, sick, sick. Everywhere. During the height of it. Terrible...the entire ER was an ICU when I got back."

March 13 was probably too late for schools to have closed in New York City. The Department of Education reported that eighty-seven school-based employees in the city had died of COVID as of fall 2021, overwhelmingly in the first wave of the pandemic before shutdown.

RELYING ON PUBLIC SCHOOL FOR FOOD, LAUNDRY, AND HEAT

One of the reasons that leaders hesitated was that New York City had so many children who relied on school for food. Of the 1.1 million public school students in New York City before the pandemic, three-quarters had qualified for free or reduced-price lunch based on family income until the city decided to simplify things by feeding all comers for free. One in ten was housing insecure.

In New York, media reported that the chancellor, the mayor, and the governor were hesitating to close schools. That was because of the extraordinarily large number of families who "rely on our public schools for more than learning, like food, laundry, and heat," in the words of Councilman Justin Brannan. Chicago and Los Angeles officials made similar statements about "our obligation to provide essential services that…students and parents depend on." In the next chapter I'll get into how schools struggled to keep feeding kids.

When schools closed in San Francisco, Jonah's parents were worried about his best friend. Khamla and Jonah had met a few years before in elementary school, shortly after Khamla, the only child of older parents who spoke no English, arrived from Laos.

"My first year of school, I have no friends," Khamla says. "My mom bought me cupcakes to bring to school and give away. When you have good stuff in your lunch, like gummy snacks, like cookies, everyone is asking you for one." Jonah invited Khamla to his birthday party, and the rest is history. Khamla often counted on Robert and Maya to help him cope with the strangeness of California life. When schools closed, Robert stopped by to make sure he had a school computer, a Wi-Fi hookup, and a grocery card to make up for the loss of school meals.

THE REFRIGERATOR GETS UNPLUGGED

In March 2020 people all over the country and all over the world suddenly understood what schools had been providing, like a giant refrigerator whose background hum you don't hear until someone pulls the plug. Public school closures went from difficult to devastating as weeks turned into months because when the buildings closed their doors, the US lost its largest, most robust piece of public infrastructure.

In the United States, there is no strong legal establishment or broad cultural understanding of a universal right to afford basic necessities like health care, housing, or childcare for young children.

But we do offer twelve years of universal, free public education, including meals and some access to health care and mental health care, to children ages five and older—even for undocumented immigrants. No one is turned away from a public school.

That's a remarkable anomaly if you stop to think about it.

Schools began as local and voluntary efforts. They have always been highly contested, subject to the whims of local politics, and relatively underfunded. Yet they persisted.

COMBATING THE "OLD DELUDER SATAN"

The first publicly funded schools in North America were founded by and for northern white settlers. They predate the Constitution by more than a century. They established some enduring precedents: schools are to be mandatory, local, funded in common, and dedicated to the moral improvement of humanity, not just basic skills.

The Old Deluder Satan Act of 1647 in Massachusetts stated, "It being one chief project of that old deluder, Satan, to keep men from the knowledge of the Scriptures, as in former times by keeping them in an unknown tongue, so in these latter times by persuading from the use of tongues," as soon as a town grows to fifty households, a schoolmaster should be appointed to teach the children to read and write.

Oh, and this early law laid down the precedent that schools should be competitively priced: "Those that send their children be not oppressed by paying much more than they can have them taught for in other towns."

The Constitution itself omitted any mention of education. This may be because the southern colonies had no such early tradition of common schools. Rich white children had tutors in the home or were sent back to England for education. Other white children labored in their own homes or others'. Not until 1705 did Virginia decree, "The master of the [apprenticed] orphan shall be obliged to teach him to read and write."

Enslaved people learned however they could, by the dispensation of certain enslavers or in defiance and in secret, as Heather Andrea Williams writes in her book *Self-Taught: African American Education in Slavery and Freedom*. Teaching enslaved people to read was outlawed because education is an essential step in the recognition of humanity and citizenship.

"I was compelled to resort to various stratagems," wrote the abolitionist Frederick Douglass of his own snatched self-education. "I had no regular teacher." These stratagems included convincing white children he met in the streets to give him lessons.

Many of the nation's founders advocated for expanding the common school system. Thomas Jefferson's Bill for the More General Diffusion of Knowledge was defeated repeatedly in the legislature of his home state of Virginia, and he concluded in disgust, "People generally have more feeling for canals & roads than for education."

James Madison, for his part, advised, "Schools for the education of all should be placed at convenient distances and maintained at the public expense. The revenues of the State would be applied infinitely better, more charitably, wisely, usefully, and therefore politically in this way than even in maintaining the poor. This would be the best way of preventing the existence of the poor."

THE FANTASY OF MERITOCRACY

Here Madison introduces an alluring and enduring bipartisan American fantasy: that it is possible to create a meritocratic economy of opportunity through education alone, rather than redistributing wealth. In this way, we can somehow "prevent" poverty in the future, rather than help the people who are already here.

Early Americans pursued education as a means to shape society, founding church and charity schools. Alexander Hamilton and John Jay were among the founders of the Manumission Society, organized in New York for the purpose of "mitigating the evils of slavery, to defend the rights of the blacks, and especially to give them the elements of an education." Manumission was a gradualist alternative to abolition. The society's school, the New York African Free School, opened in 1787 near what is now City Hall. That is, the first free school in New York City was for Black children.

"THE MICE HAVE FORSAKEN IT"

In the nineteenth century, the federal government used land grants in the western territories to help pay for common schools. Still, Washington, DC, continued to take a very minor role in funding and directing public education. This was a notable difference from other countries, where public education was highly nationalized and centralized. Up through 2020, under 10 percent of the budget for K–12 education came from Washington.

Absent a constitutional mandate or robust federal funding, schools have always been run on nickels and dimes. New York funded them with state lotteries as far back as 1799, a practice that continues in several states today. New Orleans taxed theaters; Connecticut, liquor licenses; and the nation's capital appropriated to its schools a special tax on enslaved people and dogs.

This legacy of marginal funding is embodied in the complex where Jeannie teaches and where she attended and her five children go now. The building fronting the highway, which houses the high school, is a stately but run-down graystone built by the Works Progress Administration as part of the New Deal in the 1930s. Other buildings were tacked up in the 1960s, and the latest additions are "temporary" trailers that have been up since Jeannie was in middle school in the early 1990s. She gets riled up when she drives by the prosperous cattle and chicken ranches on the outskirts of town. Her conservative neighbors refuse to vote for bonds to fix up the school.

When people complain about badly built public schools today, they are echoing complaints from hundreds of years ago. Horace Mann was an abolitionist whose résumé included founding the state's first insane asylum. In 1837 Mann became Massachusetts secretary of education, the first in the nation. He embarked on a grand inspection tour, visiting a thousand common schools on horseback over six years. He found, mostly, neglected, drafty old wrecks. "Ill-constructed shell of a building...uncomfortable seats," he reported of one building, and memorably of another, "Before the next gale is over, foundation stones would be all that remain of it....The mice have forsaken it." Out west on the frontier, schools were sometimes housed in sod dugouts or abandoned saloons.

To an astonishing degree Mann envisioned the public education system we have today. He campaigned to expand common schools, draw wealthier students away from private schools, compel students to attend school, have the state take over charitable schools, and increase local and state taxes to pay for it all. And over the course of the nineteenth century, he largely succeeded.

He pushed for the nation's first compulsory education law, passed in Massachusetts in 1852. By the year 1870, all states had elementary schools that were free to students, paid for by taxpayers, and that students were increasingly required to attend. The United States, among whites, soon boasted one of the highest literacy rates in the world.

THE END OF THE "COMPULSION" IN COMPULSORY EDUCATION

Requiring students, by law, to come to school is a simple yet revolutionary policy. We don't have laws forcing people to vote or to otherwise take part in civic life. But education is something we consider important enough to make everyone participate in some way.

Reciprocally, it's the one service the state must provide to every child. Even teenagers in jail. Even children living in cars. Even children who are chronically ill or nonverbal. Even migrant children detained at the border.

This revolutionary, reciprocal commitment was one of the first things to go away when schools closed.

I learned this from José Luis Vilson. In March 2020, Vilson was teaching middle school math in Washington Heights, the majority-Latinx Manhattan neighborhood made famous by Lin-Manuel Miranda's musical *In the Heights*. He was overseeing the education of his own eight-year-old son Alejandro at home. Vilson, who is Black and Latino, is also the executive director of EduColor, an organization dedicated to race and social justice. Like a few other teachers I know, he left the classroom during the pandemic year.

His neighborhood was hard hit by COVID. Many of his students had essential workers in their families. Vilson told me that with students out of the classroom, the "compulsory" part of compulsory schooling was, basically, gone. He had no recourse—other than the relationships he had already built—to make his students listen, learn, or do their work. "[In normal times], if I wanted to get my class to do something, 25 percent of the kids would do it without me having to ask. There's a broad swath, say, about 50 to 60 percent of the kids, who I'm constantly having to, like, poke and prod. . . . And then there's like maybe the 20 to 25 percent of kids who, they have a hard time doing it regardless of whether or not I'm on top of them."

Those kids were now coping with the stress of a pandemic and the frustration of online learning. Walking out of class was as easy as turning the camera off or wandering away from their seat. Vilson tried to improve engagement by adding riddles and nonacademic questions to his teaching. He says some of his fellow teachers "were extremely frustrated when they realized students were just saying, no, we're not doing this because we're not in school."

The 150-year-old social contract of public schooling in America—you must show up, we must educate you—was broken.

SCHOOLS AS BATTLEGROUNDS

It was foretold long before the pandemic that closed schools would hit differently in different communities based on race, class, and politics.

The expansion of public education into a compulsory and universal institution was propelled not only by progressive reformers like Mann but by ruling-class interest in schools as an instrument of assimilation and social control. The nineteenth century was a time of rising immigration, frontier battles, and abolitionist upheaval. The drive toward compulsory education met resistance from many quarters.

In the big East Coast cities, once they had to send their children to school, immigrant Catholics and Jews started to protest the heavily Protestant curriculum, which was a carryover from the old church-based charity schools. The bishop of New York City's St. Patrick's Cathedral, John Hughes, was known as "Dagger John." He thundered, "We are unwilling to pay taxes for the purpose of destroying our religion in the minds of our children."

These sectarian curriculum battles sparked nativist, anti-immigrant riots in New York and Philadelphia. New York State offered a compromise: the Maclay Bill of 1842 barred all religious instruction from public schools but provided no state money to denominational, including Catholic, schools. Dagger John retaliated by founding the Catholic parochial school system, which is still the largest alternative school system in the country.

African Americans, meanwhile, petitioned without success for the right to attend the public schools they paid for with their taxes. "These separate schools cost more and do less for the children," Black citizens wrote to the Boston School Committee in 1846. "The school rooms are too small, the paint much defaced, the apparatus is so shattered it cannot be used.... We therefore earnestly request that our children be allowed to attend schools in the Districts in which we live."

Frederick Douglass wrote in words that would be echoed by civil rights activists in the twentieth and twenty-first centuries, "The point we must aim at is to obtain admission for our children to the nearest school house, and the best school house in their own neighborhood."

Around the same time, in 1860, the Bureau of Indian Affairs established the first Indian boarding school on the Yakima Reservation in the state of Washington. These schools in name only, run by the military and the church, perpetuated abuse and cultural genocide—intended "to kill the Indian and save the man," in the infamous words of Captain Richard H. Pratt, founder of the Carlisle school in Pennsylvania.

The boarding schools have left their scars in Jeannie's corner of Oklahoma. Her ex-husband's parents met at Haskell, founded in 1884. And even today, some local kids with behavior problems still get sent to the Riverside Indian School in Anadarko, Oklahoma, founded 1871.

In 2020 mass unmarked children's graves began to be discovered on the property of residential schools in Canada, where they were mainly church run. Secretary of the Interior Deb Haaland, the first Native American cabinet member, announced an inquiry into the corresponding sites in the United States.

In short, public schools (a.k.a. government schools) have always meant different things to different communities, and the feeling they brought wasn't always gratitude. Far from it. Crumbling, underfunded classrooms; campaigns for access and against segregation; curricula condemned for its cultural erasure; none of these are new.

A public school classroom can be a site of oppression, discrimination, bullying, and indoctrination, as well as of solidarity, love, self-actualization, and collective liberation. Often they have been both. And that is why they are so hard to perfect, to control, and—until 2020—to do away with.

PUBLIC SCHOOLS HAVE CRITICS AND ENEMIES

Public schools have always had critics, like the members of marginalized groups who want them to do better, to be fairer, more democratic, more responsive, more accessible. They also have always had enemies.

The pandemic hit in the midst of a multi-decade, richly funded political effort by the enemies of public education, a movement whose most prominent face in 2020 was the secretary of education.

Opposition to public education as such, now and historically, brings together evangelical Christians (who resist public schools as a stronghold of secular humanism, feminism, and LGBTQ rights), cultural conservatives (who resist exposure to antiracism and other tenets of liberalism), corporate capitalists (who resist them as a remaining bastion of unionism), and libertarians (who resist compulsory education as one of the most significant and extensive government interventions in private life). Then there are millionaires and billionaires who see K–12 education as another "sector" ripe for disruption with for-profit and online alternatives.

In other words, the core constituencies of today's Republican Party, who are otherwise seemingly so disparate, unite on this one issue. It turns out originally it was *Brown v. Board of Education*, the Supreme Court decision in 1954 that ordered school desegregation, that brought together these strange bedfellows.

Nancy MacLean tells the story in *Democracy in Chains*, her essential 2017 intellectual history of the US Right. James McGill Buchanan, a University of Chicago–trained economist and converted socialist, seized on southern white segregationist fervor in the 1950s to establish a broad, powerful anti-majoritarian movement. MacLean writes: "What animated Buchanan, what became the laser focus of his deeply analytic mind, was the seemingly unfettered ability of an increasingly more powerful federal government to force individuals with wealth to pay for a growing number of public goods and social improvements they had no personal say in approving."

As his logic goes, it is undemocratic to make people of wealth, a minority, ante up for goods and services desired by the majority. "Better schools, newer textbooks, and more courses for Black students might help the children, for example, but whose responsibility was it to pay for these improvements?"

RESIST PUBLIC SCHOOLS, DROWN GOVERNMENT IN THE BATHTUB

Buchanan's power came from understanding that the moneyed class of white people would prefer to establish and pay for all-white private schools, rather than support the improvement or upkeep of public schools now attended by significant numbers of Black students. And if rich white people could be convinced that they were justified in no longer paying for public schools, it would open the door to resist all taxation, all public goods, and all government. Anti-tax zealot Grover Norquist memorably described the idea this way: "I don't want to abolish government. I simply want to reduce it to the size where I can drag it into the bathroom and drown it in the bathtub."

Schools were and are our largest, most broadly accessible welfare institutions. So privatizing and defunding public education became a central plank of a broader anti-majoritarian, anti-regulation, anti–social safety net, and pro–wealth holder platform. Dubbed the "Marx of the ruling class," Buchanan soon secured the Koch brothers as patrons.

At Virginia Tech and later at George Mason University, Buchanan led the Center for the Study of Public Choice. "Choice," of course, is the single most familiar word to anyone who has followed education reform conversations in the past two decades. "Choice" is the banner of the political movement that upholds the systemic inequities that teachers like José and Jeannie deal with in their classrooms every day. The agenda is to shift public school money to for-profit and private alternatives; to independently run, nonunion charter schools; or to homeschooling families directly.

This movement could have no better avatar than Betsy DeVos, who grew up in a conservative Protestant enclave in Michigan, married the heir to the Amway direct-sales billions, and as a philanthropist and lobbyist backed private, religious, and for-profit schools. She had never taught in, attended, or sent her children to a public school before President Donald Trump named her secretary of education in 2017.

During the pandemic, she diverted a disproportionate share of federal relief funds to private schools, until a judge declared her actions illegal. She also declined to direct the Department of Education to track or publish information on school reopening plans or COVID mitigation strategies, abdicating responsibility for helping districts reopen safely even as the Trump administration called for them to reopen at any cost.

Corey DeAngelis is a fellow at the Cato Institute—another Koch-funded organization, which also counted Buchanan as a distinguished senior fellow—and is one of the current standard-bearers of conservative thought. And he's the research director of American Federation for Children, a group founded by the DeVos family that advocates for vouchers and other alternatives to public school.

"One of the main problems with public schools in the US is the monopoly power that you generate through residential assignment," DeAngelis tells me. Or, in Frederick Douglass's words, DeAngelis objects that children mostly start kindergarten at "the nearest school house, and the best school house in their own neighborhood."

When I spoke to DeAngelis in the spring of 2021, he, like many anti–public school conservatives, saw opportunity in the crisis: "2021 could be the year of school choice, partially because of the teachers' unions' influence on keeping the schools closed for so long." His dream is a universal voucher program, where taxpayer funds are parceled out directly to families to spend as they wish, with no public school "monopoly." Meaning, no collectively funded infrastructure to provide education as a public good.

As Jack Schneider and Jennifer Berkshire argue in their 2020 book *A Wolf at the Schoolhouse Door: The Dismantling of Public Education and the Future of School*, the anti–public school political movement has grown in strength, taking on new guises, even as the desegregation efforts of the 1960s and 1970s recede. The solidarity established by the common school model of the northern colonies, where local families took up a collection to hire a schoolmaster, has eroded, and an entire political party favors the model that held sway in the southern colonies: children educated privately at home, by churches or charities, or however they can get it.

THE JOB OF SCHOOLS HAS CHANGED

When you think about how devastating it was to close public schools, in small-town Oklahoma, in cities like San Francisco, in places in between, it ought to raise some questions: Why do so many American children rely on public schools for something as basic as a meal? Why do so many lack computers and internet access at home? Why do the least advantaged children go to the most crumbling schools—why not target funding where it's needed most?

The critics of public education are correct that spending has skyrocketed, even as its supporters say it's underfunded. Schools are being asked to do more. Their job has gotten more complex and expensive as they've been required to provide more equitable services to a more diverse population with more varied and significant needs.

Take the Individuals with Disabilities Education Act, first passed in 1975. It guarantees all children a "free, appropriate public education" in the "least restrictive environment" possible. Fourteen percent of public school students are now recognized as having a disability. Serving them appropriately costs more money—often many times more—than serving a student without a disability.

Similarly, one in ten public school students in the United States is learning English. New arrivals to the US were once excluded from public schools or left to sink or swim in English-only classrooms. Reaching growing numbers of English language learners with specialized teaching and materials is what justice demands.

It's pragmatic: this is the future workforce. It's also more expensive.

EDUCATION ALONE CAN'T PREVENT POVERTY

US children are relatively more likely to grow up with material hardship than they used to be, compared to older Americans. And educating children in poverty, if you want to do it successfully, costs more than teaching middle-class and wealthy children.

As recently as 1989, about one-third of K–12 students nationwide came from low-income households. Welfare reform gutted support for families in 1996; the Great Recession came in 2008. By 2013, the share of public school students in low-income households crossed 50 percent for the first time.

Existing structures of inequality map onto younger generations. Today's children are the most racially and ethnically diverse generation of Americans. About half of all children today are not white, roughly double the proportion in the population at large.

Jeannie's students in Oklahoma reflect this shift. They include resettled Hmong refugees and Spanish-speaking recent immigrants. An increasing number live in trailers out on "the ranch," an unincorporated piece of property with cheap lots but no water or sewage hookups. Others are closer to town, in public housing or individual homes built or financed by the Cherokee Nation or various US government aid programs.

Before the introduction of Social Security in the 1930s and Medicare in the 1960s, older Americans were the age group most likely to live in poverty. Since then, Americans began living longer, potentially outliving their savings. Wages stagnated, and poverty overall rose.

But thanks to that monthly cash benefit and regular cost-of-living increases introduced in the 1960s, poverty among older Americans has fallen by two-thirds, and now they have the lowest poverty rate of any age group. In 2020, the age group most likely to be living in households earning below the poverty line was children.

James Madison's ideal, which you still hear repeated today, is that, instead of directly reducing poverty, we should invest public money in education—thus empowering individuals through opportunity, or in his words, "preventing the existence of the poor."

But there are diminishing returns to this approach. Rampant child poverty undermines the job of schools. This goes beyond the obvious facts of children too hungry, or too tired after a night in an overcrowded apartment or trailer home, to concentrate, or children embarrassed to come to school because their clothes are not clean.

TRAUMA AND EDUCATION

The past few decades have brought major scientific revelations about how children's early experiences shape their developing brains for a lifetime. Vincent Felitti, then head of Kaiser Permanente's Department of Preventive Medicine in San Diego, became interested in the number of extremely heavy adults he treated who turned out to have suffered sexual abuse as children. He began what became known as the first Adverse Childhood Experiences Study in 1995, with seventeen thousand participants.

Child sexual abuse, it turned out, is one of ten adverse childhood experiences, or ACEs, as Felitti called them. As he and other researchers documented, an ACE produces what is called "toxic stress." This is stress that chronically changes the mix of hormones and neurotransmitters in a way that has observable effects on the structure of the brain in critical periods of development. These changes, on average, hurt mental, physical, and emotional health—and in turn, educational attainment and earning power—for a lifetime.

Poverty itself, when it leads to material neglect, is an ACE. And it multiplies the chance of other ACEs. A child growing up in poverty is twice as likely to experience a pile-on of three or more other adverse childhood experiences. These can include a parent's incarceration or death.

This statistic tells us one stark thing. If our society doesn't divert its vast resources to lower family poverty, we are actively choosing the mental and emotional suffering of children every single day. And those early days of suffering reverberate for lifetimes, across the entire society and economy.

Well-off children experience ACEs, too, of course. Divorce, a parent's mental health struggles or substance abuse, and physical or sexual abuse are all on the list.

Could the pandemic itself be considered an ACE? Most of the experts I talked to didn't think so. A better metaphor is to think about COVID as being like the climate crisis. More heat stress, more energy going into the atmosphere raises the likelihood and the intensity of individual disasters like wildfires and floods. Those disasters, in turn, are visited most intensely on the vulnerable. In the same way, rather than think of COVID as itself an ACE for all children, it raised the background conditions that made ACEs more numerous and more severe, especially for children who are already vulnerable.

TRAUMA MAKES TEACHERS' WORK HARDER

Jeannie carried ACEs into the classroom with her as a student. Now as a teacher in the same classrooms, she sees her students struggling with them too. When she used to teach high school, the older students kept their home life bottled up, but her sixth graders open up to her about families struggling with mental illness and substance abuse.

As José Luis Vilson told me, so many of his students who resist the demands of the classroom are holding these kinds of burdens. When students are going through trauma, teachers must work hard to establish trust so their students feel safe enough to listen and are therefore capable of learning.

This changes the nature of the job that teachers like Jeannie and José have to perform every day. Their work is so much more than conveying information through intellectually engaging lesson plans. On a good day they are helping students meet basic physical and emotional needs, a role that comes at a psychic cost because the children in their classrooms inevitably need more than they have to give. And on a bad day, just one distressed child, expressing themselves in the only way they can, can bring learning to a halt for a classroom of thirty. This is a reality I've witnessed as a journalist for more than a decade.

WE KNEW, OR WE SHOULD HAVE KNOWN

In March 2020, in the United States, people in power knew, or should have known, that keeping schools closed for even a few weeks would have serious, long-term, inequitable consequences. Closing schools is nothing like closing restaurants, gyms, or offices. In a country as unequal as ours, with so many children in need, it is more like closing hospitals or soup kitchens.

And we also quickly knew something about how to mitigate the risks of keeping schools open.

In March 2020, it was apparent that COVID behaved very differently than previous epidemic diseases like polio and influenza with regard to children. This right away undermined the logic of prolonged school closures as an intervention.

Past infancy, people were less severely affected the younger they were. There still is no great explanation as to why. One prevalent hypothesis is that children's immune systems are simply better tuned to respond to novel viruses, since they are more likely to be encountering any given pathogen for the first time. A second is that they are more primed by frequent exposure to various coronaviruses, such as colds.

In March 2020, we also had some ideas about how to keep both children and adults safer when congregating indoors. A set of safety measures—masks, distancing, handwashing—were immediately improvised where necessary, such as in childcare centers that kept operating for essential workers. Experience showed that these measures reduced spread in settings where children were gathered and that compliance could be good even among young children.

These guidelines were quickly adopted by the Centers for Disease Control and Prevention (CDC). Our contact tracing was never what it should have been, but evidence mounted around the world that schools and childcare facilities could actually be operated more safely than other types of indoor gathering places like bars, restaurants, factories, or gyms—usually, when these measures were followed, with fewer cases than in the surrounding community.

The potential risks and the immediate harms of closing schools also multiplied and gathered force over time, from learning to mental health, physical health, and economic and emotional stress on families.

And yet our schools—historically underfunded and inequitably funded, governed by more than thirteen thousand separate locally elected boards, contested sites of opportunity, embraced and mistrusted from community to community—were unable to open as quickly as they had shut.

In places where schools opened in the fall, after delays and often with limited in-person days, majorities of parents kept their kids home anyway, mistrusting their safety, particularly if they were Asian American, Black, or Latinx. And, as the pandemic raged on into a third wave and then a fourth, schools closed often and unpredictably, sending many students home to quarantine.

WE STUCK OUT FROM THE WORLD

This limited, inconsistent, and unequal access to in-person schooling is one of the more damaging ways that the US experience during the pandemic stood out globally.

There is an entire genre of best-selling books about why Japan or Finland or whoever is beating the United States in education. In 2020 the answer was simple: those places all had kids in classrooms; we didn't. The US closed most classrooms for a total of fifty-eight weeks, compared with thirty-three weeks in Finland, twenty-seven weeks in both the UK and China, eleven weeks in Japan, and just nine weeks in New Zealand.

Some parts of the world, mostly in Asia Pacific, got the pandemic under control and therefore were able to reopen schools quickly and safely with a minimum of public conflict. Other places, for example, across Europe, the UK, and Israel, prioritized schools. They reopened as soon as April but certainly by the fall of 2020. They closed classrooms again as little as possible, even when infections were growing. They closed businesses, nightclubs, and other adult gathering places rather than schools and childcare. The United States everywhere failed to prioritize children in this way. The decision on opening schools was determined by political affiliation more than the local course of the disease.

There were also countries that did worse than the US when it came to both schools and the pandemic. In many lower-income countries, school closures lasted past the one-year mark, reversing hard-won recent progress in school enrollment. Combined with the global economic crash, continuous closures in places like Mexico, Kenya, Bangladesh, El Salvador, Uganda, India, and Brazil drove boys into paid work or onto the streets, and girls into paid work, domestic labor, or early marriage.

The World Bank estimated that without heroic remediation, seventy-two million more children worldwide will be illiterate or out of school entirely as a result of these closures. The setback could be devastating. For individuals' lives and dreams, for economic growth, and even for issues like the climate crisis. Girls' education in particular, historically neglected in many places, is seen as a key lever for equitable and sustainable development.

Among these diverging global paths, the United States stuck out: a rich country full of poor children, doing one of the world's worst jobs controlling the pandemic. Prolonged school closures hurt children in this country. Some were deprived of basic needs. Most lost learning time and suffered socially and emotionally. The most vulnerable were indeed hit hardest. Those losses will take time and concerted effort to overcome. And, as a painful twist, it became controversial even to say so.

It may take years to understand what our children lost because of prolonged school closures, just as it may take years to recover.

JEANNIE BROUGHT IT HOME

Jeannie is the one who brought home to me just what school closures did to families like hers. Not just practically but emotionally. She said she was being hard on herself for not coping too well in the first weeks. "I didn't have to go to work. I was at home and safe and I had everything. Nothing was bad. And I could not figure out why I was so crazy. I was so off."

And then, one day she was sitting in the car waiting to pick up Ruby from gymnastics when it hit her—the school closures were bringing her back to her childhood trauma. "I'm reliving my mom's divorces. This is what's happening. This is why I've been crazy, because there's no stability."

That flash of insight, in turn, helped her have compassion for her neighbors. Mainly they were Trump supporters. They denied the seriousness of COVID, growing increasingly impatient with teachers like Jeannie over school closures.

> We've been attacked on Facebook and social media. The parents are upset and I'm mad at them for that. I'm hurt that they would turn on us.
>
> But I also understand. Because most of the people in my area have gone through a lot of trauma as well. We're poor and uneducated. They grew up in trauma and then they put the trauma on their kids. It's just a cycle. And so their stable places were taken from them, too. And I don't want to get angry, because we didn't provide for them. We didn't provide that stable place for them this year—or their children.

2   HUNGER

So you're talking about 2.2 million deaths—2.2 million people from this. And so, if we can hold that down, as we're saying, to 100,000—that's a horrible number—maybe even less, but to 100,000; so we have between 100- and 200,000—we all, together, have done a very good job.

—Trump at a White House task force press briefing,
March 29, 2020

April 10, 2020, US seven-day average of cases: 31,709

Serena was four years old when the pandemic hit. She shared a twin-sized bed with her mother, Elisa, in a single room that rented for $1,000 a month in the Outer Sunset neighborhood of San Francisco. The kitchen and bathroom were split with two other families.

Elisa came to the United States from Peru and speaks Spanish. At the time of lockdown, she had one job cleaning hotel rooms and a second job cleaning the house of a man she called Don Victor. He fired her because he was worried about COVID exposure since she rode the bus to work. Elisa told me many of her friends who were cleaners for "Americans" kept getting paid during lockdown. Don Victor, who was Mexican, didn't pay her beyond the first week. But he did say she could come to one of his restaurants and get free food for herself and Serena.

The first time she asked for two burritos. The second time, around lunch, she asked for three. The man behind the counter called the boss and passed the phone to Elisa. "Hello, Don Victor, how are you?"

"Why are you asking for three burritos, Elisa? There are only two of you." She wept as she recalled the humiliation. "I said I was asking for one more for dinner."

CHEF ANN

Chef Ann Cooper, who calls herself the "lunch lady on a mission," runs the food program at Boulder Valley Public Schools in Colorado. An athlete with a toothy grin and a blonde crop, she once wore her toque at fine-dining restaurants and cooked privately for the Grateful Dead. Gradually, she became obsessed with school lunches and the world-changing opportunity they presented: to feed children real food from local farms, building strong bodies and healthy lifetime habits while supporting local, sustainable agriculture at a large scale.

In Boulder Valley, where I visited her in February 2020 on assignment for NPR, the kitchens were the heart of the schools. Compost barrels sat on scales hooked up to tablet computers to track food waste. Middle schoolers did their science projects on composting and competed in Iron Chef competitions to add their own recipes to the menu.

When her schools closed, Chef Ann had to change how she operated overnight. With little in the way of official guidance, she divided her staff into three crews that did not overlap, to reduce the risk of contagion. Everyone was in gloves and face masks, and sanitization protocols were running overtime.

Within a few days, her kitchens were giving out seven thousand bags of food per week. Morale was high, she told me, because her staff could see that the food was sorely needed. But at the same time, they were nervous about coming in to work when everyone else was ordered to stay home. When we spoke in April, Ann's face on Zoom was grim; the responsibility for her team's safety was weighing on her. Indeed, a California study later found that line cook was among the more dangerous jobs in the pandemic. "School lunch staff are all of a sudden becoming first responders," she told me. "And that's just not something that most people signed up for."

Despite the heroic efforts of the Chef Anns of the world, distributing meals this way just wasn't as efficient as feeding kids who were already physically coming to school. The Food Research & Action Center surveyed fifty-four large school districts and found that the number of lunches given out in April 2020 dropped by 70 percent from the year before. In October 2020, after schools had had several months to figure out the process, the figure was nearly the same—66 percent lower than the year before.

FOOD SPOILAGE

The stakes of closing public schools were never just students' academic progress. As they were scrambling to set up distance instruction plans, schools had an entirely different, enormous job on their plate: they had to figure out how to keep feeding children.

School cafeterias in the United States serve about 7.5 billion hot meals in a normal year. It's the second-biggest anti-hunger program in the country after the Supplemental Nutrition Assistance Program, or SNAP, formerly known as food stamps. Nearly thirty million children depend on free and reduced-price school meals, which include breakfast, lunch, dinner, and summer meals.

These federally funded meals actually predate food stamps by three decades. This chapter explores how that came to be—how child hunger was all but eradicated in this country over the course of half a century, thanks to anti-labor-union busybodies, staunch segregationists, the Black Panthers, early tabloid TV producers, and J. Edgar Hoover. And then, during the pandemic, how that system failed.

It wasn't for lack of trying. By the end of March 2020, school districts set up thousands of drive-through and walk-up food sites.

They spent money on new refrigerators, masks, gowns, and gloves. They used school buses to deliver meals to students, sometimes along with packets of work, laptops, and mobile hotspots, and they partnered with nonprofits to mail groceries directly to families in rural areas. They dealt with supply chain disruptions. Farmers, early on, were plowing under onions and dumping milk as they tried to cope with suddenly closed restaurants and cafeterias, on the one hand, and raided supermarkets on the other. Schools did all this while also managing their whole other job of, you know, teaching students.

At the same time, unemployment was skyrocketing. Women were especially likely to be driven out of work. And parents found it harder to work because, of course, schools were closed.

The CARES Act (for Coronavirus Aid, Relief, and Economic Security) passed March 27, 2020. When the rug was pulled out from under families across the country, when the economy was put in a medically induced coma, there was an openhanded response from a Republican president and Republican-controlled Senate. Near-universal cash payments. Enhanced unemployment benefits. More SNAP money to households already in the deepest need. There was also a program meant to send the cash value of school meals directly to families. It was called Pandemic Electronic Benefits Transfer (P-EBT); SNAP benefits are typically loaded onto prepaid debit cards.

But help took time—in the case of P-EBT, over two months for the first installment and several more months for the second. There was red tape and there were gaps. State unemployment agencies were overwhelmed by the demand. Undocumented immigrants sometimes felt unsafe signing up for benefits.

Households with children, and particularly Black and Hispanic households, went hungry, especially in those early days, at rates that hadn't been seen in a generation. Around 30 percent of households with children reported food insecurity from April to November 2020. That was double the rate in 2018. And it was ten points higher than the rate for households without children.

WAITING IN LINE

Into the void left by institutional and government aid stepped a huge amount of mutual aid and charity. Free food fridges popped up on street corners, and shuttered restaurants were repurposed as food pantries. These efforts were necessary and innovative and lauded. They could also be stigmatizing and complicated and exhausting to access. Elisa found it so excruciating to be browbeaten by her ex-boss that she never went back to the restaurant. With Serena in tow, she spent hours waiting in line at various churches and food pantries.

Patricia, in DC, and her husband have lived in her car. They know what it's like to need assistance. During the pandemic she was tireless in support of her community. Her actions were in line with research that suggests the lowest-income 20 percent of Americans are twice as generous, proportionately, in charitable giving as the top 20 percent.

She helped organize giveaways of food, tampons, diapers. She picked up donations from a nonprofit called Martha's Table to help her neighbors, including the elderly relatives of the woman who ran the daycare Patricia's older son, PJ, attended. Patricia also donated from her own household, even though the family was getting behind on bills, as there was less money coming in from her side jobs: refereeing local rec sports games and delivering for DoorDash.

Helping out this way, being face-to-face with people's needs, can be difficult for both the giver and the receiver. It was an invitation to judgment, because in the United States, dignity and basic survival are not generally understood as rights guaranteed to everyone. They are linked, and have been for centuries, with some idea of moral worth. Those who don't meet a shifting set of expectations can be left to fend for themselves. Maybe that link is especially vivid for someone like Patricia, who was raised in foster care.

At Thanksgiving, Patricia told me, "It made me feel some type of way about people, because they seem very ungrateful. We gave this one lady a turkey and she was like, 'Oh, no, I want that bigger one right there.' And I looked at her and I said, 'Ma'am, this is free. You need to take this or you can get back in line.' And then [her] little girl said, 'Mommy, we already got to several other places.' And I just kind of looked at her."

On the other side of the breadline might be a woman like Sheila. As a single mother out of work in the East Village, dealing with long-haul COVID symptoms, with three hungry teenagers at home, she found herself swallowing her pride and going to food pantries for the first time in her life. Once a church turned her away because she wasn't a member. Sometimes the lines were two hours long. Her father is Cuban, but Sheila presents as white. She imagined people looking at her and wondering, "What is this white lady doing here?" She also had her own assumptions about the people joining her in line: "You stand on the queues and you feel uncomfortable because it's either, you know, homeless people, sometimes drug addicts."

Receiving charity face-to-face requires a specific emotional performance on both sides that isn't there in the same way when you pick out exactly the cut of meat you want and swipe a benefit card at the grocery store, or when you sit down in the lunchroom with your classmates, all of you with the same tray of hot food and carton of milk.

SCREAMING INTO THE VOID

Between April 23 and May 19, 2020, one analysis found, food insecurity doubled overall and tripled among households with children. While 30 percent of households with children were food insecure, the figure was 41 percent for Black and 36 percent for Hispanic households with children.

In another survey, four in ten mothers of children under twelve reported household food insecurity in the first few weeks of the pandemic, and 17 percent said their children were actually not getting enough to eat.

There is an important distinction here. Food insecurity, the broader measure, includes buying less meat, reducing portion sizes, switching to canned vegetables from fresh. For Elisa it meant paying the rent instead of buying groceries; even though there was an eviction moratorium in San Francisco, she didn't want any debts.

Like other kinds of insecurity, food insecurity is a mental state, too, one of worry and preoccupation. Elisa was shorter-tempered with Serena than she would have liked. She was too tired to read to her or help her with her schoolwork.

Hunger is different. It means actually skipping meals, running out of food at the end of the week, going to bed hungry. "I could have died from hunger," Elisa told me. "I was eating just things that I had left in the house." Serena had been a picky eater, fond of candy, and now there was no way to get her favorite things.

As they saw these numbers coming in, hunger researchers and advocates felt like they were screaming into a void. Economist Diane Schanzenbach is a star in the world of child benefits. She's done groundbreaking research on the introduction of food stamps as part of the War on Poverty in the 1960s and 1970s, demonstrating that it improved birth weights and lifetime health outcomes for children with access to the program before the age of five. And for little girls in particular, there was also a measurable impact on life outcomes: those with access to food aid as children were more likely to graduate high school, earned more, and were less reliant on public benefits as adults.

"Why is it not penetrating the discussion?" Schanzenbach asked me about family hunger when we spoke in December 2020.

You know, as an economist, I want the world to be rational, and I just cannot understand what is going on here. These are just levels that we've never seen before. You know, usually we study this broader measure, which is food insecurity, and do less on hunger [itself] because the rates are so low that most data sets don't have enough sample rate.

Now one out of six adults with kids is saying that [the kids] don't have enough food, they're actually *hungry*.

This indicated an extraordinary situation of need, researchers told me, because typically older family members will skip meals themselves before they let children go to bed hungry.

Lauren Bauer, an economist at the Brookings Institution, was equally outraged. "This is not a fun thing to be working on right now. I have a PhD and I generally do research on kids. And at least since the pandemic started, as a mother myself, I have the brain capacity to deal with one issue in my portfolio, and this seems like the most important one. And I've completely ignored almost everything else that I do research on, just to focus on dealing with hungry kids."

Bauer's experience was not unique. More than nine out of ten of the researchers, advocates, and other experts I talked to for this book were women. Because that's who tends to study children. And a great number of those women were raising children themselves. At the time when the country needed voices like Bauer's the most, their capacity was limited by the same catastrophe that was affecting everyone else.

"It would be my strong preference that we didn't have to get this bad for people to take action," Bauer continued, "because I think normally, you know, we sort of have an agreement that kids in the United States should not be hungry. And in normal times, our combination of programs gets you close. It's not perfect. But, normally, not only do the federal nutrition assistance programs and the safety net prevent kids from experiencing hunger but their parents too." These programs taken together, she said, provide about half the calories consumed by poor children in America.

HUNGER PANGS

Even when hunger lasts a short time, the harms can linger for decades. Pregnant women who aren't well nourished have babies who weigh less and struggle more to survive. And as Schanzenbach told me, birth weight has been studied extensively as an indicator of lifetime health outcomes and social markers, like high school graduation rates. Hunger in young children is associated with chronic illness and behavior problems, as well as lower school performance, attendance, and grades.

Chronic malnutrition, a lack of essential nutrients, is believed to interfere with brain development. Food insecurity, the preoccupation with having enough, is associated with high levels of parental stress, and therefore with mental health problems and behavior problems in children.

Sheila lives in a rent-stabilized apartment in the East Village. In 2020 she had seventeen-year-old twins and a nineteen-year-old in special education. She worked in marketing in the travel industry and was laid off on April 2. The date sticks in her mind for two other reasons: "It was my thirtieth anniversary with the company. And the day I found out I had COVID."

She wasn't hospitalized, but serious fatigue lingered. "You go outside, you'll start to go for a walk and everything feels heavy. Like your eyelids are heavy. Your hands are heavy. It's heavy to move your body; it's a little labored to breathe. And it's just like, OK, I'm going to push myself because there's one store and then I get to go back home." She wasn't able to look for work for months.

"This is so hard, to come to a food line and ask for help. It's not how I was raised; it's not how I was taught. I'm from a lower-middle-class family; my mom at least always had mac and cheese and apples. We had nothing else, but she always figured it out. And I have three kids on my own, so I had to figure it out." And she always did, until the pandemic.

Sheila said that one of her daughters became depressed during the pandemic. "We had to put her on meds. She can't get out of the house." For teens, old enough to understand the struggle to stretch groceries through the end of the week, food insecurity has a particular association with mood, behavior, and substance disorders—over and above poverty alone. Teens report forgoing food so that their younger siblings can eat or trying to stay away from home during meals.

The impact of hunger can be surprisingly long lasting. Tragically, studies of the Dutch "hunger winter"—a wartime season of extreme deprivation caused by the Nazis in Holland in 1944–1945—actually seem to show an epigenetic impact. That means that the hunger appeared to affect genetic expression for babies in utero during this time. Most strikingly, that generation grew up to have a higher risk of schizophrenia.

Ending hunger should be a social priority. It's the fundamental human need. And hunger in children, from infants to teenagers, has reverberating effects.

Investments in children, like any long-term financial investment, bring compounding returns. Harms to children have long-term consequences.

Hunger is one need the United States was doing an OK job of meeting before the pandemic, at least compared to other children's needs, like housing, health care, childcare, or mental health. Our failure here is especially heartbreaking. It was, as Bauer points out, predictable from the structure of this disaster. "Households with children are more likely to go hungry. That's always the case when there are economic interruptions. It is more the case now for a couple of reasons."

First, school closure meant a loss of childcare. Second, and in part as a consequence, women lost most of the jobs during the COVID recession. For both of those reasons, single-mother households like Sheila's and Elisa's were particularly hard hit. And they were at the bottom of the economic ladder already. Third, school closure meant a loss of access to school meals.

In the previous chapter I discussed the strange historical accident of how free, nonsectarian public schools became not only available but universal and compulsory in a nation without much of a welfare state. I think it's worth looking briefly at how we got to the combination of programs Lauren Bauer is talking about—the history of making sure children are fed, both inside school and outside of it. It was a long, arduous process undertaken by people with multiple and sometimes contradictory instincts and motives. And the progress is especially instructive as we think about what kind of social effort can produce a better country coming out of this disaster.

CHILDREN OF THE TENEMENTS

We left off our school tale in the previous chapter in the mid- to late 1800s, when public school was made compulsory for the first time by state laws across the country. Enrollment skyrocketed. An increasing number of the new students in big cities were newcomers to the country as well. Between 1880 and 1920, twenty million immigrants from eastern and southern Europe came to the United States, joining previous waves from Ireland, Germany, and China. Poverty was high in these communities, as documented by muckraking photographer and author Jacob Riis. His publications, with titles like *The Children of the Poor* (1892) and *Children of the Tenements* (1903), focused particularly on the plight of the young, including "newsies" working in the streets and the inhabitants of orphanages, asylums, and day nurseries.

Socialists and labor organizers fought for industrialists and elected leaders to combat this poverty by redistributing wealth and property or, failing that, raising wages. The wealth holders themselves, not surprisingly, had other ideas.

Edward Atkinson was not your average fat cat in a top hat. He was a hardcore abolitionist—a supporter of John Brown—and an active anti-imperialist. He was also a cotton mogul, with mills throughout New England, and a fierce defender of the wonders of capitalism.

Atkinson published his book *The Science of Nutrition* in 1896, after his workers went on strike. At the time he calculated that all but the wealthiest 10 percent of Americans were spending about half their income on food. His goal with this book was to prove that a man could eat for no more than twenty-four cents a day, at a time when average wages were $1.50 a day. And so, you see, there was no need for him to raise wages! Instead, the housewives of working men should be instructed in substituting lard for butter and beans for meat.

Atkinson followed principles first developed in feeding livestock to break food down into basic elements like protein, carbohydrates, and fats. *The Science of Nutrition* also included a design for what he called the "Aladdin oven," essentially a slow cooker, to tenderize cheap cuts of meat with minimal fuel. Andrew Carnegie, fellow white-bearded captain of industry, loved the book so much he put a copy in each of the public libraries he established at that time around the nation.

Just like today's billionaire philanthropists, Atkinson hastened to found a social enterprise to put his theories into practice. Together with Mary Hinman Jonah and Ellen Richards, two of the founders of what became known as home economics, Atkinson opened the New England Kitchen in Boston on January 1, 1890. As described by culinary historian Barbara Haber, items like beef broth, cornmeal mush, pea soup, Indian pudding, and oatmeal cakes were offered for takeaway for just fifteen cents a meal. The enterprise failed commercially, reportedly because the Jews, Portuguese, and Italians in the North End weren't big fans of mush. But Richards negotiated with the Boston School Committee, a volunteer group of parents and philanthropists, to pivot to producing and delivering meals to the city's high schools. Within a year five thousand students were eating soups, sandwiches, meat pies, scalloped potatoes, cakes, and puddings at school every day: the nation's first school lunch program.

School lunches grew from there. In some places, "mothers' clubs" fed hungry kids. Other schools ran lunch programs at a profit. The growth of school lunch coincided with the establishment of home economics in schools. In fact, sometimes the school lunch program *was* the home economics program: girls were trained to cook and their meals sold cheaply to fellow students.

SCHOOL LUNCH POLITICS

Gradually, taxpayers were convinced to ante up for hungry kids. Child hunger became a national security issue when one-third of First World War recruits were rejected for physical problems like rickets. A 1918 study estimated one in four children was malnourished. From World War I through mid-century, according to Susan Levine's 2010 book *School Lunch Politics*, volunteer parent and teacher groups sponsored "weigh-ins" of schoolchildren. Just like prize livestock, the biggest gainers were lined up at the front of the class. They got gold stars or a yellow balloon that read "good health." One congratulatory note read, "Anna Carado keep it up, Anna you're a dandy / Don't forget the milk and fruit and leave alone the candy." Teachers discovered that when hot lunch was served, children came to school more often, paid more attention, and behaved better.

The Great Depression brought yet another spike in child hunger and malnutrition. In 1936, children on average weighed less than they had five years earlier. This was the point when the federal government first got involved in school lunch.

Franklin Delano Roosevelt's New Deal propped up Big Ag in many ways. It excluded agricultural workers from both the Fair Labor Standards Act and Social Security, and extended credit to large farms. In 1933 the nonprofit Federal Surplus Commodities Corporation was formed to buy up agricultural surpluses, serving as a price support for farms. Only then did the idea arise to distribute the purchased food to school lunchrooms. As administrator Marvin Jones put it, "Everyone liked to see children well fed."

To get the food, the feds required communities to provide matching funds and hire permanent staff, including professional nutritionists. Strict nutrition requirements were written into these contracts, as they are to this day. President Roosevelt tapped none other than legendary anthropologist Margaret Mead to create the first Recommended Daily Allowances. She determined that all seven food groups, as she identified them, must be included in each school meal: green and yellow vegetables; oranges, tomatoes, grapefruit, raw cabbage, and salad greens; potatoes and other vegetables and fruit; milk and other milk products; meat, poultry, fish, or eggs, or dried beans, peas, nuts, or peanut butter; bread, flour, and cereals; and butter or fortified margarine.

In 1936, federally subsidized school lunches fed 350,000 children a day. By 1942 the number was more than 5 million, or about 1 in 4 schoolchildren.

The law also asked schools to serve free meals to the poor and treat all students equally. Fat chance. There was no enforcement, little oversight, no local matching funds in places like Texas and Virginia, and very few free meals for Black kids in particular.

By 1943 the New Deal was over, and the lunch program was set to phase out. A Coordinating Committee on School Lunches formed— a national citizen effort to "save the school lunch program." A Mrs. Harvey W. Wiley, representing the General Federation of Women's Clubs, testified in 1945 that without free food, free education was wasted: "If education is given free in the public schools, then food must now be given to enable the hungry children to absorb the education provided, or else it is thrown away."

SWEET MILK AND SOCIALISM

The 1946 bill to create a permanent school lunch program was co-sponsored by two segregationist southern Democratic senators: Allen Ellender from Louisiana and Richard Russell Jr. from Georgia. Not coincidentally, they were two heavily agricultural states.

If Russell's name sounds familiar, it might be because the Senate office building is named after him. He was a mentor to President Lyndon B. Johnson and served for decades. And he used his mastery of Senate rules and procedure to block civil rights legislation for much of that time.

Opponents of the idea of a federal school lunch program attacked "unnatural mothers" who wanted the state to raise their kids. Amazing phrase! We'll hear it again when it comes to childcare in the next chapter.

These opponents were also interested in impressing on children at young ages that, well, sorry, but I have to do this: there is no such thing as a free lunch. They were worried that budding capitalists might be corrupted by "the idea that you can get something for nothing from Uncle Sam."

In the summer of 2021, a school board member in Waukesha, Wisconsin, put forth a very similar view. Karin Rajnicek said that if the district were to continue offering free lunches to everyone under a pandemic-era federal program, children might "become spoiled."

Back then, Senator Russell countered that hot lunches were good for democracy. "In my opinion a school child who has a good bowl of hot soup and a glass of sweet milk for his lunch will be much more able to resist communism or socialism" than the one who has a hard biscuit in a tin pail.

The National School Lunch Act passed on June 4, 1946. The program was structured primarily as an agricultural subsidy administered by the Department of Agriculture with no involvement of the federal Department of Education; it remains so today.

One congressman declared he'd never seen so much support from people "from one end of the country to the other—regardless of race, creed, or color." That may be so. But the moralizing and discriminatory nature of the program persisted for yet another two decades, until the federal government was shamed into expanding the program by the scariest activists, and some of the most audacious advocacy, some people had ever seen.

HUNGER IN AMERICA

In May 1968 viewers across the country watched an American baby die of malnutrition on national television. The shocking sequence occurs in the opening minutes of *Hunger in America*, a nationally televised special on CBS that may be one of the most effective pieces of policy propaganda ever produced by the US news media. It was one of the key contributing factors to finally producing an effective free lunch program.

The 1960s saw a new national conversation about poverty and child hunger, one that finally incorporated a whisper of justice and equity. "In the last year we seem to have suddenly awakened, rubbing our eyes like Rip van Winkle, to the fact that mass poverty persists, and that it is one of our two gravest social problems. (The other is related: While only eleven per cent of our population is non-white, twenty-five per cent of our poor are.)" That was Dwight Macdonald writing in the *New Yorker*, in an influential review of Michael Harrington's even more influential 1962 book *The Other America*. The book, a document of poverty in the midst of plenty, is credited in part with inspiring President Lyndon B. Johnson's War on Poverty.

Free school lunches were mandated in 1962 as part of that War on Poverty, which also introduced food stamps. But there was no federal funding to back up the free lunch mandate for four years after it first appeared. That came with the 1966 Child Nutrition Act.

Federal War on Poverty programs required a national standard for determining who was poor. So it was that in the mid-1960s, home economist Mollie Orshansky invented the federal poverty line. She made up a model "thrifty" food budget and tripled it, reasoning that the average family spent about a third of their income on food. These days that assumption is way off; families spent just 9.5 percent of their budgets on food in 2019. Other necessities, like housing, education, and health care, are relatively much more expensive than they were more than a half century ago. So the federal poverty line—$17,420 in 2021 for a household of two—is now considered too low to give an accurate estimate of how many are living in real deprivation.

By the 1960s, the school lunch law was fairer than before, but practice still trailed the law. Activists—both reformist and revolutionary—were important in pushing the government to live up to its promise.

The Committee on School Lunch Participation formed in 1968. Advocating on behalf of hungry children, something civic-minded mothers had been doing for decades, was less controversial than advocating for equality for women or Black adults, so it drew many mainstream liberals who might have been scared off by other causes of the times.

The committee sent representatives in neat suits and hats to lunchrooms across the country to produce the 1968 report *Their Daily*

Bread, underwritten by the Field Foundation. This report made clear why the federal government needed to take further action to guarantee equal access to free school lunch. In some places, they reported, Mexican American children were expected to take out the trash and clean the school bathrooms in exchange for a lunch token. School leaders judged individual children and their families on deservingness. "Look at the fat arms and muscles," an educator said of one child in Florida. "That kid's all right." Children in West Virginia were reportedly denied if their fathers were known to be drinkers. One family was taken off the "free list" because they had a television at home.

Hunger USA, a second report published in 1968, was also funded by the Field Foundation. This report became the basis for the CBS documentary. It was filmed in historical bastions of poverty that are still all too familiar today: the black belt of Alabama; the barrios of San Antonio, Texas; and the Navajo reservations of Arizona.

To a present-day viewer, the tone is both condescending and exploitative. We hear about hungry children living in homes with a "late-model television" and "empty pint bottles." There are lingering shots of crying, underweight babies, skin wrinkled from dehydration. On the Navajo reservation we see the gums of a child bleeding from scurvy and hair that is reddish from a lack of protein, a disease called kwashiorkor. We see tiny burial mounds in the cemetery, belonging to children who starved to death.

Senator George McGovern was among the viewers at home. In one scene, a child told the presenter, Charles Kuralt, that he did not have the money to buy a school lunch and felt ashamed. McGovern reportedly turned to his wife and said, "We are the ones who should be ashamed, and I am going to do something to change this."

SURVIVAL PENDING REVOLUTION

One other group was crucial in getting free school lunches funded: the Black Panther Party. Bobby Seale and Huey Newton met as students at Merritt Community College in Oakland, California, and founded the group in 1966. While they've long been caricatured as violent militants, the Black Panthers' legacy is being reconsidered lately in light of the Black Lives Matter movement, for example, in the Oscar-winning 2021 film *Judas and the Black Messiah*.

There's more attention these days to the group's mutual aid and direct action work, which Newton called "survival pending revolution." It included a network of free clinics, a school, and the Free Breakfast for School Children Program that first opened its doors at St. Augustine's Episcopal Church in Oakland. From 1969 through the early 1970s, the program expanded to forty-five sites across the country and fed tens of thousands of hungry children. In fact, it fed more children in the state of California than the school lunch program was managing to do at the time, an accomplishment that was noted in a 1969 Senate hearing.

Considering the many decades of "mother's clubs," teachers, and other women engaged in the necessary work of feeding hungry kids, it's enormously refreshing to see the photos of Panther men, with Afros and golf caps, handing out chocolate milk, eggs, meat, cereal, grits, toast, and fresh oranges to children holding up the Black Power fist in salute. The program fed all comers, with no eligibility tests, no weigh-ins, and no shaming. "The children, many of whom had never eaten breakfast before the Panthers started their program," one newspaper wrote, "think the Panthers are 'groovy' and 'very nice' for doing this for them."

You know who didn't think the Panthers' breakfast program was so groovy? J. Edgar Hoover. Because of its popularity, and the positive reception among both white and Black moderates, the FBI director singled out the Free Breakfast program for ire. He called the program "potentially the greatest threat to efforts by authorities to neutralize the BPP [Black Panther Party] and destroy what it stands for." Hoover had, apparently, allies in the police department in Chicago. "The night before [the first breakfast program in Chicago] was supposed to open," a woman Panther told historian Nik Heynen, "the Chicago police broke into the church and mashed up all the food and urinated on it."

The Free Breakfast program declined with the systematic harassment, repression, and arrests of Panthers around the country. But public pressure and grassroots efforts were finally coming to a head in Washington.

George McGovern and Senator Bob Dole, his colleague across the aisle, introduced legislation in 1970 that funded free and reduced-price school meals at new levels. Some of the money was used to build kitchens in city schools that had none.

The program expanded along with food stamps, a lunch program in childcares for younger children, a summer food program, and a special milk program for women with babies.

Thanks to a combination of volunteerism, business initiatives, propaganda and political activism, and an unlikely coalition of radicals and moderates working over decades, several generations of babies managed to grow up in the richest country on the planet without too many of their families worrying about them dying of starvation or suffering diseases of malnutrition.

All of this worked so well that the most recent authorization of the school lunch program, the Healthy, Hunger-Free Kids Act of 2010, was focused on childhood obesity, micronutrient deficits, and access to fresh fruits and vegetables, not stunted growth, rickets, or bleeding gums.

It worked so well that visionaries like Chef Ann dared to dream of a school meals program that leveraged its scale and historical connection to the US Department of Agriculture to not only feed children but build community, improve farming practices, and actually grow a better, healthier planet for kids.

And we might still get there, but in 2020 we went backward: to Sheila in New York and Elisa in California, bodies aching from COVID and from work, standing in line for hours outside of churches and warehouses, with hungry mouths to feed at home.

3   CHILDCARE

So, supposing we hit the body with a tremendous—whether it's ultraviolet or just very powerful light…supposing you brought the light inside the body, which you can do either through the skin or in some other way, and I think you said you're going to test that, too. It sounds interesting. And then I see the disinfectant, where it knocks it out in a minute. One minute. And is there a way we can do something like that, by injection inside or almost a cleaning. Because you see it gets in the lungs, and it does a tremendous number on the lungs. So it would be interesting to check that.

—Trump, April 23, 2020

May 12, 2020, US seven-day average of cases: 23,677

Habersham is a Black boy with apple cheeks and dreamy eyes. In the spring of 2020 he is seven years old. He stays most of the time with his mother and seven siblings in half of a duplex apartment on a blocked-off street strewn with garbage in St. Louis. Plastic bins of clothes, toys, kitchen gear, and other belongings are piled high in the window wells of their home, blocking the light. There's a broken-down van parked outside the house, with more clothing and toys crammed inside. At the end of the block there's a view straight to the Gateway Arch.

Habersham likes animals. He begged his mother for a kitten. When it gets hot out, he goes looking for fireflies in the many vacant lots in the neighborhood. He likes to cuddle his baby brother and two little sisters. He's closest to his next-oldest brother, Shadrack, who's twelve and has a sly sense of humor. He also has some teenage siblings, who stay sometimes with them and sometimes elsewhere.

Heather, Habersham's mother, is petite and stylish, with a broad smile like her son's and pastel-colored hair that sometimes cascades past her shoulders. Her Facebook feed is a stream of inspirational quotes and affirmations: "Don't be pushed by your problems. Be led by your dreams." "You may not be where you want to be, but you're not where you used to be." Positive thinking is key to Heather's survival, but it's not always easy. Her world is divided into friends and enemies, upturns and downturns of fortune.

When COVID hit, her fifteen-dollar-an-hour job as a certified nursing assistant ended. She found another job at a homeless shelter. But she had a problem. The daycares in her neighborhood had closed because of the pandemic. "There were no outlets—no places for them to play. None of the centers were open."

This was a common problem: two-thirds of childcare centers closed in April 2020, and one-third remained closed even in April 2021.

The older kids watched the little ones. Fathers, cousins, family friends pitched in. But when she had to go to work, Heather sometimes resorted to locking the door on the younger children for a few hours.

Habersham didn't spend much time on school; there weren't enough working computers or space to use them at home. But he found a profitable way to pass all his new free time. He would put on his red school uniform polo shirt and khakis and dodge the traffic to get over to the Family Dollar store, where a cousin worked. There, looking like a little store employee in uniform, he would hold doors and carry bags for tips. When he got some money, he'd go to the corner store and buy a hot meal, like ravioli or ramen, in a Styrofoam cup.

In the late afternoon of May 12, 2020, Habersham ran off with some older friends. The boys broke the window of a nearby building and climbed in. A man inside shot him in the leg and his twelve-year-old friend in the wrist.

Heather's throaty voice catches as she remembers rushing to the scene. "There was a lady already helping my baby and several police officers. I was about to pick him up and put him in the police car because the ambulance wasn't coming. I was totally distraught. I couldn't believe that my seven-year-old son got shot in his leg. I just wanted to be there with him, be there for him." Heather says the building was vacant, being used as a "trap house" by drug dealers. The newspaper called the incident an attempted burglary and referred to seven-year-old Habersham as a "suspect." No one pressed charges.

Habersham recovered, but Heather remained without childcare.

CHILDCARE IN TATTERS

Heather's situation was extreme. But in that first spring of the pandemic, millions of parents all over this country felt the loss of a trustworthy pair of hands to help care for their children while they worked for wages and did the other tasks that keep life running. With almost every school and after-school program shut down, a large chunk of childcare centers closed, and extended family less available because of COVID exposure worries, parents ran out of options. Or, to put matters another way, even upper-middle-class families were suddenly staring into the abyss of care that less wealthy parents had been dealing with all along.

"It's a disastrous system, if you even want to call it a system. It's awful for children. We need revolutionary change," according to Kimberly Morgan, a political scientist at George Washington University. That's a view shared by every single person I talked to who knows anything about childcare.

The problem is this. The United States makes no effort to provide for childcare as the public good that it is. Other rich countries have guaranteed paid family leave, childcare subsidies directly to families, and publicly funded childcares. Before the pandemic, average annual public spending on early childhood care across rich countries was $14,436 per child. In the US it was $500. Lynette Fraga, of the organization Child Care Aware, told me that childcare was, if anything, becoming even more inequitable and inaccessible in the years before COVID. The average cost of center-based care *doubled* from 1999 to 2019. The number of providers was dropping in most states. Half of the US population now lives in what Child Care Aware calls "deserts of quality," where there are three or more young children for every spot in a high-quality program. The geographic distribution of high-quality centers is important, Fraga told me, because childcare, like politics, is local. "Traveling twenty, thirty, forty, fifty miles to a childcare program is obviously not doable for families."

CARE COSTS MONEY

Good childcare is expensive. There are no real economies of scale and no acceptable shortcuts. The younger children are, the lower the ratio of children to each caregiver should be. Nurturing a growing human is best done by someone with extensive training or experience, ideally both. Children bond with their caregivers; they need stability, but low wages usually mean high turnover. If only for our children's safety, we would like their caregivers to earn a living wage so that they can work reasonable hours and come to work calm, well fed, and rested. And maintaining a healthy, safe, and inviting environment, with a recently disinfected changing table, toys, books, not to mention fresh air and outdoor space—all of that costs money too.

So care for young children is not some kind of mass-produced commodity that the market can provide affordably by driving down the margins. It's also not a great candidate for gig work. You don't want to push a button on an app and have some nearby stranger come to your house to stay with your toddler. Because of these inherent realities, quality childcare must be publicly subsidized, by paying family members to stay home or paying for outside providers, typically a combination.

Here in the United States, with our meager public subsidies, three things happen. Quality goes down. Care becomes unaffordable for most families. And simultaneously it becomes a poverty-wage job for almost all providers. Child Care Aware reported in 2020 that the cost of full-time center-based care for two children ranges between $18,442 and $26,102 a year, depending on the region—more than housing, food, or anything else in an average household budget. Yet the workers in those centers were making about $25,000 a year.

THE LASER MAZE OF CARE

Now that more, and especially more privileged, Americans have experienced an interruption in childcare, the sector has seen more focus than it has for decades.

In the spring of 2021, President Joe Biden seriously proposed mending the tatters, even weaving some new cloth.

But we've been here before. In the 1940s and again in the 1970s, Uncle Sam got so, so tantalizingly close to providing broad childcare benefits before pulling back. And sometimes the very people you'd think would be the biggest champions of childcare have let down the cause.

The politics of childcare are complicated.

The whole field is crisscrossed with bright lines and third rails, like one of those laser mazes in a heist movie. People, especially mothers, who want to stay home with their own children and be paid for it have sometimes found themselves at odds with those who want childcare provided by others so they can work. The cold logic of the market divides the (mainly) women who provide domestic labor from the (mainly) women who purchase it. And educators have created and policed a boundary between them and mere "babysitters," a boundary that sometimes gets them more resources and respect but doesn't necessarily serve children.

The pandemic may have ratcheted up the urgency and started a new conversation. But putting our hands on the big jewel—a world where all of our children are cared for lovingly and safely—is going to ultimately require unwinding a lot of attitudes ingrained for centuries about gender, race, and the true nature and importance of care work.

So let's break it down. Here in the twenty-first century, three-quarters of all parents work for wages, most of us full-time. We don't have a national program of paid family leave—the only country among the forty-one "most developed nations" without one. So families need someone to watch the children while they work, for at least, say, the first thirteen years of their lives. That comes out to twenty-seven thousand hours of care, assuming a forty-hour workweek.

CHILDCARE BIOGRAPHIES

I asked Heather in St. Louis, as well as Dara in New York, Jeannie in Oklahoma, Patricia in DC, and Maya in San Francisco, for their childcare biographies. Their stories show how parents with different resources and circumstances cobble together their options—with ingenuity, hard work, and the generosity of community.

Heather's, and at certain points Jeannie's, children qualified for Head Start, the free, federally funded program for children under five. On the whole it's really decent. But it's for families below the poverty line. And the federal poverty line, as mentioned in the previous chapter, is way too low. It's just $18,310 in 2022 for a household of two. Notably, Head Start eligibility is far lower than food stamp eligibility, which goes up to 185 percent of the federal poverty line in most states. Therefore, the reach of these programs is limited: they serve just 820,000 of the twenty-three million children under five in the United States.

The vast majority of Head Start centers closed as of March 24, 2020, and remained closed in many cases throughout the spring and fall, leaving the neediest children in the country without childcare. Thanks to their federal funding, their staff did continue to get paid and were assured of reopening, and like public schools, these centers worked hard to provide their enrolled families with meals, remote programming, and connection to other services like housing.

All of the mothers I followed took advantage of free, informal help at times. More than half of all hours of nonparental care for children are unpaid, according to the Urban Institute. This includes care by extended family, friends, and neighbors. Asian American, Latinx, and recent immigrant families are more likely than others to live in intergenerational households, which makes for easier access to grandparent care. Care from loving extended family can be wonderful, but it's not always available, and there's little opportunity for regulation or oversight. The pandemic interrupted many of these arrangements because older people were more vulnerable to the virus. In other cases, grandparents moved in. The pandemic brought a big jump in multigenerational households, with 34 percent in one survey saying that childcare was the main reason for the new arrangement.

Another free resource all these families used over the years was public school and public preschool. As parents discovered during the pandemic, one important function of public school is to provide a safe place for children to be for six or seven hours a day.

Jeannie has run the gamut of childcare options with her six kids, the five she is still raising and the first, who was born when she was a teenager. "With my oldest, he went to daycare his first year. Tennessee paid for that because I was still in high school. Then we moved back to Oklahoma, and my grandma kept him while I worked and went to college. With Julian and Rob, they went to daycare, and I paid out of pocket. With Ruby, their dad lost his job when she was a few weeks old, so he stayed home with her until she went to school. He started working night shift at his current job at the Tyson feed mill and kept her and the twins during the day."

Jeannie is rare in that her kids' dad was the primary caregiver, even briefly. George, her ex, told me the time he spent with his girls was "excellent.... I really bonded with them." National polls find that before COVID, fathers were spending just eight hours per week on average directly on childcare, against mothers' fourteen.

When Jeannie and her husband divorced, she qualified for daycare help for the twins from the Cherokee Nation, a Head Start program, and Oklahoma's free public pre-K. When COVID hit, George was still sharing their house and helping out where he could. But his job at the feed mill was considered essential, and he worked long hours, starting at the crack of dawn, six days a week.

Jeannie says that her mental health wasn't the best during this time: she was staying up late scrolling through the news and the occasional conspiracy theory on Facebook. She checked out at home and stopped enforcing many rules or routines. Julian, the oldest, was working at Sonic, and Rob, at thirteen, mainly stayed in his room playing Xbox.

That left Ruby, at ten years old. She both played with and watched her eight-year-old twin sisters daily. "We [she and I] are the hub of the household," Jeannie wrote to me. "I did not place her there. She stepped in, and I am incredibly grateful but also incredibly sad for her."

Ruby was not alone. Across the country, and around the world, girls in particular took on more care responsibilities when schools and childcare shut down, sometimes at the expense of their own studies and their mental health. Like Ebony, a sixteen-year-old I spoke to in New Orleans, who had moved out of her mother's house to live with a friend and found herself supervising Zoom school for half a dozen children. "They're running around screaming every morning. They have the most energy! I would cook for the kids. I had to be with them in the kitchen and sit everybody down, make sure that they had what they needed. It wasn't just me making sure that I was on my Zoom call. I had to get these meeting passwords for all their teachers too. It was very overwhelming."

Patricia in Washington, a connector by nature, has also called on a village of family, friends, and paid care over the years. She had her older son, PJ, in July 2015, several weeks early, and was back working in a DC public school classroom by August. A woman named Miss Chris, who was Patricia's good friend's mother-in-law, watched baby PJ at her house for a while, until her own grandbaby was born. When PJ got older he attended DC's universal public pre-K and after-school programs.

For her younger son, Patrick, she was diligent and savvy enough to get a childcare voucher. These subsidies, paid for by city, state, and local governments, reach just one in six eligible families. And the quality of care varies. "People think I was crazy for sending him to a daycare in Ward 8," she said. "They say it's ghetto—that's not my opinion, it's just what people think. I haven't had any issues with it." When school started again in the fall of 2020, she sent PJ, now a kindergartner, to a home-based provider called Gifted Academy. Patricia made up the fees partly by helping the operator get school supplies, computers, and other donations through her school district and neighborhood connections. Theresa Garza, the founder, helped PJ with his remote learning so Patricia could do her own work helping *her* students with their remote learning.

In-home group providers offer the most affordable paid option in childcare. These small businesses, which are exempt from some licensing requirements, took care of seven million children, including around 30 percent of all infants and toddlers, before the pandemic. Across the country almost all of these providers are women, and almost half, like Garza, are women of color.

Jessica Sager teaches a seminar on childcare and public policy at Yale and is the founder of All Our Kin, a national nonprofit organization that helps provide equitable access to quality childcare through teaching, training, and supporting family childcare educators.

Sager is passionate about this army of caregivers. She calls them "really the backbone of our childcare system." These centers, she told me, are conveniently based in the neighborhoods where parents need them. They speak people's languages, and they provide familiar food and culture. Parents of infants and toddlers, especially, often prefer the warmth of a home setting. The centers are also often the ones who give the overnight and odd-hours care that is increasingly necessary for the children of precarious shift and gig workers.

But home-based care has historically gotten no respect, even by the already-maligned standards of childcare. Sager tells me:

> I would walk into a meeting with policy makers at the state or the national level, and I would say, "I'm working with family childcare educators. They are providing wonderful care for children. How are we going to be including them in our professional development streams? How are we going to be including them in our funding streams? They're connecting children to health care—how are we thinking about that?" And folks would look at me and say, "You are talking about babysitters who sit at their kitchen table talking to their friends while the TV goes all day long?" Absolutely blatantly incorrect statements by people who had never set foot inside of a family childcare home.

Maya, in San Francisco, was a single mother by choice until she got together with Robert when Jonah was six. Her mom pitched in a few hours a week to give her a rare break, and so did another woman from her mother's commune.

Jonah's preschool teachers were the first to help her realize that he needed interventions and evaluations that would eventually lead to diagnoses of ADHD, autism, and dyslexia. "They asked me, how do you handle him by yourself? There are three of us! And they just loved him. Jonah has always been lucky enough to have teachers who really loved him." By the time of the pandemic, Maya was more comfortably middle-class. She had Jonah enrolled in public school, an after-school program, and special activities like parkour. Because she could pay for private tests and evaluations, Maya also was eventually able to get a behavioral therapist who met with Jonah every afternoon after school through dinnertime and even on the weekends. Fifteen hours a week was covered by insurance.

Maya's also in a tax bracket that enables her to use the federal dependent care tax credit of $6,000. The credit is not refundable. That means it's regressive: it benefits higher earners like Maya, who have greater tax liability, more than the poor.

Dara, the New York City doctor, was at the top of the ladder not only economically but in social capital. Of the families I followed closely throughout the year, only Dara still had two parents who were alive, and willing and able to care for her three children for as long as a few weeks at a time. She also represents the sliver of Americans who can actually afford full-time childcare even in an emergency.

For years, with Dara working long hours at the hospital and her husband in finance, her family has hosted au pairs, a program that has its own special labor law and visa status. Au pairs come from another country and are supposed to work no more than forty-five hours per week. In exchange they receive room, board, and $4.33 per hour in cash wages.

Valencia, Dara's twenty-four-year-old au pair, joined the family from Mexico in January 2020. "It was a cultural shock—a big change for me," she said. And then her life was upended all over again.

Valencia had little control over the fact that she was living in the home of an essential worker who treated COVID patients. Instead of comparatively light duties shepherding children to and from school and activities, she found herself presiding over full days of Zoom school. Instead of spending weekends out with new friends, she was on lockdown with her employers, all of them going through stress and grief. She couldn't return home for more than a year or see her boyfriend in Seattle. She lost some members of her family in Mexico, including her ninety-three-year-old grandmother, to COVID.

Still, Valencia told me she had it a lot better than other au pairs. "I actually heard from other girls that the parents, as soon as they got nervous about COVID, they start getting rid of girls. And some others have been working for a lot of extra hours, and they aren't getting paid." There have been accusations of abuse and mistreatment in the au pair world for years, just like elsewhere in the underfunded, disrespected, shadowy caregiving economy.

"A lot of things have happened to her over the past year. And she's actually handling it really well," said Hannah of her au pair. "I have a lot of respect for her. She's, like, pretty cool."

THE HISTORY OF CARE WORK

Disparaged when they are not invisible, care workers are often triply marginalized by race, class, and gender. Women of color represent 20 percent of the US population but 40 percent of all childcare workers, according to Child Care Aware.

These patterns go back a long way.

In the time of slavery, Black women were exploited as domestic caregivers with ruthless disregard for their own family bonds. Katie Sutton, a woman born into enslavement and interviewed by Works Progress Administration researchers in the 1930s, recalled, "When I was a little gal, I lived with my mother in an old log cabin. My mammy was good to me, but she had to spend so much time at humoring the white babies and taking care of them that she hardly ever got to even sing her own babies to sleep."

The historic bias hardly ended with the Emancipation Proclamation. In fact, it was encoded into law by the domestic service exemption from the Fair Labor Standards Act passed as part of the New Deal. Other kinds of workers scored new protections under that law. But from 1938 until 1974, employers were not required to pay housekeepers, maids, cooks, or nannies minimum wage or overtime. And to this day, so-called casual babysitters are still not required to be paid minimum wage—a carve-out in the law that's big enough in practice to drive a truck through. They can also be hired as young as twelve years old, another exception to federal labor law. Live-in domestic workers, similarly, are still exempt from overtime requirements, for no good reason except that their employers prefer it that way.

Isolated in the homes of their employers, domestic workers are harder to organize than other workers, although groups like the

National Domestic Workers Alliance have lobbied successfully for more legal protections in certain cities in recent years.

Today US immigration policy continues to ensure an ever-present pool of off-the-books domestic workers. They come from Central America, Southeast Asia, the Caribbean, the Himalayas, West Africa. With language barriers, working out of public view, they are especially vulnerable to exploitative wages and working conditions—all the way to the extreme of being trafficked to this country and placed into what the State Department calls modern-day slavery.

THE COST OF LOW-COST CARE

Our tattered system hurts caregivers. And it hurts children. Too many babies, whose brains are growing faster than they will ever again in their lives, spend their formative hours and days in less safe, consistent, and enriching places, with less well-trained, well-rested people. And too many parents, overwhelmingly mothers, scale back their ambitions and earning potential. Or they compromise, with misgivings, on care that doesn't truly feel good enough for their babies.

That was the status quo prior to 2020. The pandemic made everything worse.

HOPE DAY SCHOOL

The pandemic didn't just reveal the injustices and inadequacies of our childcare system. The pandemic itself was a shock further weakening that system. Cori Berg made clear both how crucial and how forgotten these essential workers were when the storm hit.

Berg is the director of Hope Day School, a church-based childcare center in Dallas. She has round cheeks, pink lipstick, and purple-framed glasses. In a Facebook video posted in late March 2020, she is sitting in front of the altar in her church. Stained glass shines behind her, and she's surrounded by potted plants, cozy pillows, and colorful blankets. "It's Tuesday, and Tuesday is normally chapel day. And I'm by myself! So I thought I'd bring chapel to you wherever you are." She starts fingerpicking her guitar and singing: "I'll be waiting for you to come to this place. . . . Wherever you're from, I'll be glad when you come."

In this early pandemic video, Berg is doing exactly what she's done throughout her twenty-five-year career as an early childhood educator and caregiver—projecting calm and safety. Her warmth travels right through the screen. You'd never guess she was going through one of the most difficult periods in her life.

Berg's program accepts infants through five-year-olds. It's close to Parkland Hospital, which is where President John F. Kennedy was rushed after he was shot in 1963. Berg realized right away that they would need to stay open to serve the many children of doctors and nurses who attend her program. She also worried about her workers' livelihoods if they were to shut down. Caring and dedicated as she is, she is a poverty-wage employer. "I think the whole pandemic brought to light all the issues that we have had all along. . . . You know, most centers, unless they're a public program, the employees are paid very low wages. Most of my workers do not have a bank account ready to take over if they didn't work for a few weeks. And I knew that if we shut down, we wouldn't be taking in tuition. So that was part of our decision to stay open."

In the early days of lockdown, she and some of her staff worried about being pulled over on the road on the way to work. It was that unclear: Were they essential workers or not? "What was shocking was that once we started having some of the orders coming through in different counties, childcare was never actually listed as an essential worker. It would be additional language . . . oh, yes, childcare can stay open. So it was just kind of a slap in the face."

Public schools were closed, but daycares were still open. Berg said, "Many of us are like, what about our safety? Doesn't it matter? Is there going to be some kind of hazard pay?" There wasn't. In fact, because they had to reduce capacity, most childcare centers and in-home providers were working for less revenue than before. "More than anything else, it was really just feeling invisible. And that's hard when you are such a key service to every single industry there is."

Once she had determined they should stay open, Berg started looking for public health guidance on how to do so safely. There wasn't much. "I scoured the internet for resources for early childhood, and I was just shocked that nobody was stepping up to help. Not even the big names, none of our big governing or licensing bodies. This is still in March, right? There was just nothing for childcare. And yet we were really being encouraged to stay open. It was really shocking. It was terrifying."

EMERGENCY CHILDCARE

It was another example of how the US pandemic response failed to center the needs of children and their families.

Childcare providers had to improvise.

In March and April, the streets were quiet except for the sound of ambulances. I would leave my home in Brooklyn to jog or walk once a day. One morning I encountered a strangely normal sight on the otherwise empty corner: a school crossing guard at her post. From chatting with her, both of us in our masks, I realized that there were children going in and out of my local elementary school, just like before. And a few blocks away, there was an in-home daycare center where I also saw children being dropped off in the morning. I started to wonder how everyone was faring.

Starting at the moment of shutdown, the YMCA opened eleven hundred emergency childcare sites around the country, serving a peak of forty thousand children of front-line and essential workers at the height of the pandemic. As a large national organization, it worked directly with the CDC to come up with guidelines that included temperature checks, masks, and limiting group size to "pods" of ten children. It ran these programs with state subsidies at very low cost to the public.

Without its revenue from fitness centers and the like, the organization lost more than a billion dollars during the pandemic.

New York City similarly kept 170 school buildings open, including the one on my corner. They were staffed with Department of Education employees. Some came out of retirement to help, at unknown personal risk. These Regional Enrichment Centers cared for about ten thousand New York City children in March through June. They consulted with New York City Health and Hospitals and adopted rules very similar to the YMCA's. Other cities, like Los Angeles, maintained similar programs.

Berg, as an independent operator, didn't have the kind of speed-dial access to health authorities that the YMCA or the city of New York did. Her community needed guidance, so she got to work. "And probably for two or three weeks straight, I just barely even slept because I was reading everything I possibly could. Luckily, I have some connections with some other people in other states who kind of passed me little bits and pieces, and I was able to put together some protocols and think it through and start sharing those with other people—across different countries too....We had no idea what we were really doing."

She started posting videos on Facebook to help fellow caregivers figure out how to keep changing diapers and cuddling children safely.

"I just said, you know, I'm not a pandemic expert. I'm just a director like you, and this is how I'm doing it." She started with the nuts and bolts of preventing COVID spread. Here's how to disinfect wooden toys. Here's how to hold babies, facing outward and nestled against your body to limit the exchange of breath. Here's a downloadable cartoon poster that shows preschoolers how to put on a mask.

In some ways, no matter how careful they were, it all felt futile. "There's no way that you can care for children without touching them and without them touching each other." Children under two weren't able to wear masks. And caring for young children, like working in a hospital, inevitably involves bodily fluids.

Berg and other childcare providers I spoke to were understandably freaked out about their safety, especially at first. Ani Angel Gharibian, who runs an in-home daycare center in Los Angeles, told me she found the decision to close schools while allowing childcares like hers to stay open "confusing." "Schools are much larger. There's more space for the kids being distant from one another." Her voice halted as she talked about the risk to herself and her two staff members. "People are desperate for income at the moment. So even if they do have some reservations, priorities take over."

SAFER THAN IT APPEARED?

A unique study by Walter Gilliam at Yale's Child Study Center suggested that childcare centers' improvised protocols, combined with the inherently lower risks of young children catching or spreading COVID, did keep them relatively safe.

Gilliam used state registries to contact fifty-seven thousand licensed childcare workers, located in all fifty states, Washington, DC, and Puerto Rico. He tracked them for the first three months of the pandemic in the United States. During that time, about half, like Berg and Gharibian, continued caring for children under six, while the other half stayed home because their centers were closed. Controlling for demographics, the study found no difference in the rate of coronavirus infections between the childcare workers who went to work and those who stayed home.

As the pandemic raged on, there were reported outbreaks associated with childcares, but they remained rare compared to locations like restaurants, bars, gyms, and even high school sporting events.

Gilliam's study covered a time period when testing was low in the United States and so was the overall case rate outside of places like New York City. Still, the very large numbers in the study were reassuring to Gilliam, who also pointed out just how careful the providers were. "These childcare providers were doing nearly Herculean things in order to keep these babies safe. We're talking about three-quarters of them were doing temperature and symptom screenings on every single child and adult every single day. Ninety-seven percent were disinfecting all the surfaces. Over half of them were disinfecting every surface and every fixture three or more times a day. That's just incredible when you think about it."

The apparently low risk didn't change the fact that the pandemic made childcare providers' jobs even harder than before.

LOVE AND CARE

Through the early months of the pandemic, Berg put up many videos, posts, and webinars about providing the social and emotional support that children and, frankly, families and other caregivers desperately needed during this scary time. These videos are a document of the inherent tenderness of this work.

> Practice your mask expressions in the mirror so you can smile at a child with your eyes.
> Use American Sign Language signs to elaborate on your emotions.
> Say out loud, "I am feeling happy that it is almost time to go outside and play"; "I am feeling sad that it is raining right now."

In a May 12 video that made me tear up, Berg sings a song with a little girl called Avery. She asks her:

> "What do I have on my face?" "A mask."
> "What do you have on your face?" "A mask."
> "And masks are one way that we're kind to each other, OK? We keep each other safe."

She tells her Facebook audience: "You see she brushes up against me a lot, and normally I would wrap my arms around her, but for now we just kind of lean and that suffices emotionally.... It's not perfect.

But it's better than nothing. And she and I are both having fun. And we both feel safe."

THE LASTING BLOW

In the early days of the pandemic, many families' childcare arrangements fell apart. On the provider side, the whole sector suffered an economic blow that threatened to reduce, in a lasting way, the already dwindling and inadequate supply of childcare in America. The invisibility of care as an essential function of society extended to the invisibility of care as an industry.

Nearly half of childcare facilities nationwide were closed in early April 2020, according to one survey. Those that stayed open, like Berg's, were barely getting by, with severely reduced capacity and revenue.

The CARES Act included $3.5 billion in supplemental funding for childcare programs, plus another $750 million for Head Start. Airlines, by contrast, received about $13 billion in that bill. Oh, and air*ports* got another $10 billion.

Childcare providers were supposed to be eligible for small business loans under the Paycheck Protection Program, on top of direct federal aid. But many are nonprofits, and others are home based, both factors that made it complicated to apply. These PPP loans were often expedited to banks' preferred customers. In all, only about 7 percent of registered childcare businesses actually got one of those loans, representing less than half a percentage point of all the money given out. Nannies and babysitters paid off the books were at the mercy of their employers.

Texas passed an extended childcare assistance benefit for frontline workers, but the reimbursement amounted to about half of Berg's regular tuition. And her clients—the same nurses and doctors who had been paying her full freight before—weren't allowed to make up the difference. So she had fewer kids overall and was getting less money for some of the kids she did have. "In those first few months when people were getting laid off, you have your staff that you're trying to just keep paying so they can pay their bills and feed their kids and all of that, and then you have parents who are paying high tuitions. You're caught in the middle, and you're kind of the bad guy to both of them. It was just really, really tough."

CARE HAS NO PUBLICISTS

Pretty much every media outlet in the country has a food or restaurants section. Those dedicated reporters churned out thousands of articles and segments about the plight of restaurants and bars during the pandemic. And by summer, restaurants had gotten $9 billion of PPP money, compared to $2.3 billion for childcare. Childcare just didn't draw the same notice.

By June, childcare centers were reopening. But they were under conditions, like reduced capacity, that providers said could put them out of business permanently. "You know, those of us in the field, we can see centers shutting down," Berg told me. "And you're like, oh my gosh, people don't see it coming."

Sager said the first few months were devastating for the in-home providers she works with. "I think there has been a real dearth of information, a dearth of supplies, and a dearth of funding. And there is a desperate need, as any child advocate will tell you, for federal relief that just has not been forthcoming. It's actually been really heartbreakingly disappointing to see how that relief has not come through."

CHILDCARE IS INFRASTRUCTURE

Then something strange happened. People with power started to name what had been invisible for so long. On August 19, 2020, Massachusetts senator Elizabeth Warren spoke as part of the virtual Democratic National Convention for presidential candidate Joe Biden. She filmed the talk in an empty early-childhood classroom.

She reminded her audience, "Childcare was already hard to find before the pandemic." And she said, "It's time to recognize that childcare is part of the basic infrastructure of this nation—it's infrastructure for families."

What would it mean to treat childcare as infrastructure? Why haven't we done so yet?

Chapter 1 talked about the anomaly of our public school system in a country without much of a social safety net. The story of childcare is different. There's this giant, jury-rigged structure that parents and all of society depend on—from the Montessori schools, to the vacation Bible camps, to the karate dojos, to the grandmas and great-grandmas and neighbor ladies who keep extra lemonade and cookies on hand. And nobody noticed until pieces started falling off and conking people on the head.

"Children are always kind of, you know, the last bucket of consideration in public policy in the US," as Anna Johnson put it to me. She holds dual degrees in developmental psychology and public policy, and studies the impact of publicly funded early care and education on children's development. "So it's really: How can we get parents to work? How can we increase economic independence? How can we reduce the load on the public benefit system? And then kind of secondarily or tertiarily someone is like, oh yeah, maybe we should be doing something with kids."

CARE AND SOCIAL CITIZENSHIP

To better understand how we got here, there was one crucial person to call: Sonya Michel. Michel is preeminent as a historian and critic of America's careless system of care. It's a field she discovered by living the problem. In the 1980s, she had remarried, and she and her new husband were both getting PhDs—hers at Brown, his at Brandeis. "I had two older kids from my first marriage. But my second husband and I wanted a child. And I was almost forty. It was now or never. So I had a baby in graduate school. But when you're in graduate school, you're living on a pittance." They managed to get teaching assistant positions at Harvard that came with free housing in the dorms, which was the only way they could afford Cambridge's excellent—but very expensive—childcare centers. "My husband was very, you know, a New Age man, and he was very involved in helping take care of her and stuff. But notice how I used the word *helping*."

Michel didn't hold out much hope that fathers or other partners could ameliorate the caregiving dilemma by sharing the load. She put forth a more essentialist view of parenting, at least as practiced by heterosexual couples. "I think it starts with breastfeeding," she says of the typical imbalance between mothers and fathers. "You have to really make a very concerted effort to have a division of labor that involves the husband, the father."

In the society we have, childcare, Michel argues, is a particularly feminist necessity. It provides women something called "social citizenship"—that is, it allows us to participate in public life, not just in paid work. By allowing mothers to reclaim our time, public childcare "tends to neutralize the discriminatory effect of motherhood on women."

But not in the United States, it doesn't.

DAY NURSERIES AND DAME SCHOOLS

This dilemma dates to industrialization and the growth of wage labor outside the home. When people mostly farmed or worked in cottage industries, their main concern was keeping children safe and out of the way. The earliest "childcare" was provided by pieces of furniture—cribs, cradles, baskets. Many different Native peoples across the North American continent used cradleboards and slings. Puritans had "standing stools" for toddlers. When they got less portable, small children were cared for by slightly older siblings, elderly relatives, and others who couldn't do heavier work.

Enslaved people and indentured domestic servants were the preferred childcare options for middle- and upper-middle-class white people through the nineteenth century. A more affordable option for centuries, as it is today, has been women who watch a few children in their own homes. In the colonial era these arrangements were known as "dame schools."

As it turns out, what was probably America's first recognizable childcare center was founded in the wake of an epidemic. A young Quaker woman named Anne Parrish established the Female Society of Philadelphia for the Relief and Employment of the Poor in 1795. The original mission was to help women widowed by the yellow fever epidemic of 1793 with employment in a sewing workshop, plus a nursery to keep the children while they worked.

The Female Society of Philadelphia became the template for charitable "day nurseries" established in cities during the nineteenth century. They were private, targeted those deemed "deserving," and always inadequate to the need.

"Mainly they tried to just keep the kids off the street, keep them clean and keep them fed, keep them warm, so they wouldn't be endangered while their mothers were working," Michel observes. "They were pretty stigmatized. I mean, no middle-class person would be caught dead putting her child in a day nursery unless she was absolutely forced to. This goes back to the assumption that mothers should not work, mothers should be at home taking care of their children." Eligibility for day nurseries followed the four Ds: they were open to women whose husbands were disabled, drunkards, had deserted them, or died.

Wealthy, usually white women ran these programs as personal crusades. Michel quotes the sociologist Thorstein Veblen, arguing that Victorian women's philanthropy of this kind was a socially acceptable means of displaying their husbands' wealth. These women were at the top of the social hierarchy, and their children were cared for at home by domestic servants.

The problem was, the day nursery benefactors had a profound ambivalence about what they were doing, because they sentimentally preferred mother care.

When I think of Victorian motherhood, I think about "hidden mother photography." These were portraits of babies and small children taken with the long-exposure cameras of the time, which required their subjects to keep still for long periods. Someone is holding the baby, typically the mother. But that person is concealed behind a dark piece of fabric. The effect can be eerie, macabre, or absurd. Sometimes the child is surrounded by a black ghost in the shape of a mother. Sometimes only the mother's head is draped. In others, the mother can be seen off to the side, crouching behind a chair, holding up the child.

Something I've never seen explained is why the photographers, and the families who commissioned the portraits, were so determined to isolate the small child within the frame and erase the mother. This was the time of the ideology of the "angel in the house." Children were sentimentalized and adored. Domestic servitude was considered a woman's highest calling, and virtuous women were supposed to be entirely self-abnegating.

MATERNALIST POLITICS

Sociologist Theda Skocpol has dubbed the politics of Victorian childcares and other family-focused charities "maternalism"—sort of a nanny state that is, however inconveniently, anti-nanny.

Take someone like Jane Addams, who founded Hull House in Chicago in 1889 and, with it, the so-called settlement house movement, where philanthropic women lived in working-class neighborhoods both to offer services and to build community across class lines. I always admired Addams since I first read about her in high school. She was a kind of proto-feminist, both living out her own ambition and committed to other women's self-determination. Hull House offered legal aid; employment help; a nursery and kindergarten; cooking, sewing, and English classes; and even highbrow cultural programming. Addams and her colleagues lived among the women they were working with, as community organizers would nearly a century later.

But as she witnessed the struggles of impoverished immigrants, Addams began to fret that the day nursery was a "double-edged implement," that it might tempt women to "attempt the impossible"— to be "both wife and mother and supporter of the family." Michel also quotes Addams's Hull House colleague Florence Kelley wringing her hands: "No money earned in the United States costs so dear, dollar for dollar, as the money earned by the mother of young children."

It's hard to support women's self-determination if you hate the idea of them operating in the public sphere.

Michel argues this maternalist ambivalence kept the privileged women who founded day nurseries as a philanthropic pet cause from pushing them as a public policy. Florence Kelley, along with Lillian Wald, founder of New York City's Henry Street Settlement, lobbied President Theodore Roosevelt for the creation of a federal Children's Bureau, which came into being in 1912. Kelley observed that the federal government spent far more ensuring the health and growth of cows and pigs than the health of children. The first head of the Children's Bureau, Julia Lathrop, yet another Hull House alumna, was also the first woman ever to lead a federal agency.

THE CHILDREN'S BUREAU

We have arrived at a historical fork in the road. Conceivably, Lathrop's Children's Bureau could have established a national subsidized day nursery program. After all, there was a model day nursery set up at the Chicago World's Fair in 1893 that was bright and clean, charging just twenty-five cents a day to fairgoers.

Instead, Lathrop initially focused on matters like infant mortality, health education, orphanages, juvenile courts, and desertion. These were social problems largely attributable to poverty. Yet the bureau wasn't, then or later, tasked with setting up childcare so families could support themselves by working. This pattern would be repeated throughout the twentieth century and into the twenty-first: the government sees its responsibility as policing or regulating poor families, not helping them.

MATERNAL INVENTION

In the end, most working women who couldn't afford domestic servants or dame schools and who had no family to help made do without charity day nurseries and the judgment that came with them. Michel praises what she calls "maternal invention"—making a way out of no way.

For example, a lot of what was called "child labor" by progressive reformers was actually more like Take Your Child to Work Day—every day. Mothers brought children along to the seafood processing plant or the garment factory because they had nowhere else safe for them to be.

Child labor reform was another early cause taken up by the Children's Bureau in partnership with maternalist women's groups around the country. While it clearly saved lives, it also denied destitute families their children's small earnings and pushed their mothers out of the workforce, sending some children to orphanages.

Michel notes that employment rates, and the proportion of breadwinners, were always higher among Black women. This led to both a greater need for childcare arrangements and a less sentimental, or judgmental, attitude about them. The National Association of Colored Women (NACW) set up its own network of urban day nurseries for Black children. These were supported more directly by their communities, through fundraisers, for example, than the centers for white children were.

In an 1899 speech in Chicago, Mary Church Terrell, an Oberlin graduate and cofounder of the NACW, urged her fellow members to devote themselves to the establishment of kindergartens and day nurseries. She didn't say what a pity it was that so many Black women were wage-earning mothers with large families dependent upon them for support. She said, simply, "Establishing day nurseries is clearly a practical charity, of the need of which there is abundant proof in every community where our women may be found."

STARTING IN KINDERGARTEN

Day nurseries weren't the only childcare game in town in the nine-teenth century. So the story goes, at a party in 1859, a highly cul-tured and intelligent woman in the upper echelon of Boston society, Elizabeth Peabody, met Margarethe Schurz, the wife of a Wisconsin politician. Peabody was apparently really impressed with Schurz's lit-tle girl, Agathe. She remarked: "That child of yours is a miracle—so child-like and unconscious, yet so wise and able, attracting and ruling the children, who seem nothing short of enchanted."

"No miracle, but only brought up in a kindergarten," said Mrs. Schurz.

"A kindergarten! What is that?"

"A garden whose plants are human. Did you never hear of Froebel?"

Friedrich Wilhelm August Froebel, that is, the German inventor of the kindergarten. We can credit him with the 170-year enduring fad of inscrutable wooden toys painted in primary colors.

Peabody was elated. She was an abolitionist and the first woman to host a Transcendental Club meeting. She had published Henry David Thoreau's writings, translated Buddhist sutras, and studied Greek under Ralph Waldo Emerson. Now she had found her life's work.

By the next year Peabody had opened up her own English-language kindergarten, the first in the United States. She went to Germany to observe the original model and traveled the United States stumping for the idea and training teachers.

The early-education visionaries who founded kindergartens, and a few decades on, Montessori schools and other "infant schools," were completely right about some things. They were right that young chil-dren, including babies, are learning and making new brain connec-tions rapidly, and that they can benefit from a positive and enriching environment, gentle discipline, and loving care.

But the infant schools and kindergartens also entrenched the divide between what's called education and what's called caregiving.

Not only is the overall supply of childcare limited. Not only do people of all genders and all political persuasions continue to moralize and wring their hands over mothers who have other things to do with some of their time besides cuddling babies. The nation historically also divides childcare into two halves. Compared to caregivers, those known as educators get more training, higher pay, more respect, and more public support.

Early-education programs, to this day, tend to cater to wealthier parents. They have shorter hours, sometimes meeting for just a few mornings a week, and often ask for a parent to be on hand to observe or participate, a difficulty for people who work for a living.

This artificial division between childcare (no respect) and education (a little respect) is also one that public school educators reinforce. It should not be controversial to say that one important function of our public schools is to give millions of children a safe place to be during the day for free. This is an invaluable service for working parents and thus for our economy and society. But most schools maintain daily and yearly schedules that don't match the workday: six-hour days, frequent holidays and vacations, and of course, summers off. This forces parents of younger students to make up gaps with odds-and-ends solutions.

And teachers resent being conflated with lower-status childcare workers. This May 2021 tweet from Randi Weingarten, the president of the American Federation of Teachers, one of the nation's two large teacher unions, makes that attitude clear: "I think many people who saw teachers as glorified babysitters got a reality check this year when schooling had to be done at home." It should be possible to extol the hard work of teaching without disparaging caregivers. Actually, I'm on board with glorifying them.

Zero- to three-year-olds are forming brain connections at a faster rate than they ever will in their lives. They thrive on direct, focused attention and emotional constancy, and their care is physically demanding as well. How is the work of first steps and first words less important or complex than that of, say, reading or calculus?

AT THE SHIPYARD

After the Children's Bureau, the next major juncture when we could have gotten a public daycare program, but didn't, was during the Second World War. Men were sent to the front, Rosie the Riveter to the factory. From 1940 to 1945, the proportion of US jobs held by women jumped from 27 percent to nearly 37 percent.

The *New York Times* reported in 1942 that at least one desperate mother had left her child locked in the car while she went to work. That year the Lanham Act funded the Federal Works Agency to provide group childcare centers in areas of "war impact."

These centers looked after more than half a million children over the course of the war. Some were racially integrated; others were segregated, with about 260 serving only Black children. They ranged from dingy church basements to big, splashy, purpose-built projects like the one at a shipyard in Portland, Oregon. Classrooms radiated out from a central playground. The first shift ran from 7:30 a.m. to 5:45 p.m.; there was a swing and a graveyard shift as well. There was even a canteen where tired moms could pick up hot meals to take home. The total cost? Seventy-five cents, about $11.50 per child per day in today's dollars.

This working mothers' utopia didn't last long. War over, men back to work, women from coveralls into circle skirts. Federal funding for these centers shut off by 1946. In New York City mothers protested the closures with a car parade. The authorities were openly hostile. "The worst mother is better than the best institution when it is a matter of child care," declared Mayor Fiorello La Guardia. And the city's welfare commissioner, Edward E. Rhatigan, called the complainers—wait for it—"hysterical."

He sneered that a working mother earns "too little to be worthwhile at too great a cost to herself and her child" and suggested that if women couldn't manage to support their children without subsidized childcare, "extreme situations might require that the child be sent to a foster home."

Just as the federal Children's Bureau in the 1910s decided to focus on orphanages and juvenile courts instead of day nurseries, 1940s officials expressed a clear and persistent US government preference for taking children away instead of paying for care so families could stay whole.

IF NOT NOW, WHEN?

In the early 1970s, the nation had yet another kick at the Charlie Brown football of childcare. That was when Senator Walter "Fritz" Mondale, a liberal from Minnesota, introduced the Comprehensive Child Development Act. He was building on the success of Head Start, which had been introduced as part of the War on Poverty just a few years before.

The proposal was for a national network of federally funded childcare centers open to all families on a sliding scale. "Because the focus was on children...I assumed this would not be a controversial bill," Mondale recalled. Hahahaha, that's a sweet thought, guy.

It was the dawn of second-wave feminism. Women were streaming into the workforce. The National Organization for Women (NOW) was ascendant. So why did this proposal fall flat?

Anna Danziger Halperin, a historian at the New-York Historical Society, has done some provocative work on what happened. NOW's advocacy for the Child Development Act was limited in part by budget; these were volunteer-run organizations using the boss's phone lines and copy machines after hours.

But Danziger Halperin argues, based on the record, that NOW's lobbying for childcare was ultimately "half-hearted." That's because mainstream, primarily white, feminists had their eyes on a different prize. "There really is the push toward eliminating glass ceilings, and employment, and then that turns into a focus on professional women's economic success," she told me.

In our unequal system, it's mainly highly educated dual-career couples who can afford to buy their way out of the caregiving conundrum. This is actually easier to do when caring remains undervalued in the marketplace. The winners of the game don't need public subsidies. Conversely, a movement by childcare workers for better pay could actually make it harder for many working women to afford them.

It's easy to understand why second-wave feminists didn't want to overidentify their movement with women's traditional roles as mothers. Pushing for public childcare as a major feminist cause at that juncture, when the pull toward "compulsory motherhood" was still so strong, would have been like conceding that the kids are a mom's problem to solve and always will be. These women wanted exactly what men had: the privilege to pursue a career without having to worry about who was watching the children.

But just as in the nineteenth century, with the maternalist politics of day nurseries, the outcome is the same. Women with more economic and political power are choosing not to leverage that power in the interests of women with less of it. Children suffer.

THE RIGHT TO STAY HOME

During the early 1970s, the National Welfare Rights Organization (NWRO), led by Black women like Johnnie Tillmon, had yet a different focus that's also worth considering here. For centuries Black mothers have been forced to work, often at the expense of taking care of their own families. Rather than lobby for childcare, NWRO called for a "guaranteed adequate income" to allow mothers to stay home with their own children.

There was also an offshoot of the civil rights movement, exemplified by Black women–led organizations like Marian Wright Edelman's Children's Defense Fund, that successfully backed the expansion of Head Start and other programs to empower poor families in particular.

But universal childcare as a political issue remained, no pun intended, orphaned. And it remains so today.

MORAL AUTHORITY

The Comprehensive Child Development Act passed both houses of Congress. But President Richard Nixon vetoed it in 1971. He said he did not want to "commit the vast moral authority of the National Government to the side of communal approaches to child rearing over against the family-centered approach." See that word "communal"? Sounds kind of like "commune." Or "communist."

Following Nixon's lead, Republicans through the '70s, '80s, and '90s successfully demagogued any major childcare expansion as a threat to the traditional family and racialized it as a handout to "welfare queens." Often Democrats joined them. In a 1981 Senate floor speech, for example, none other than Joe Biden declared it "bad social policy" to allow benefits for "married couples who neither have the financial nor physical need to put their child in a day-care center."

That word, "need," says it all. By that logic, childcare should be a last resort, for example, if your husband deserts you, drinks, is disabled, or dies.

And that kind of tight-fisted, compulsory motherhood logic gets us directly to the nonsystem we have today.

COLLECTIVE CARE

So here is the $500 billion question.

Did the pandemic cause a large enough upheaval in the social order to change how we collectively think about care?

People stood on the street every night for months and banged pots and pans for health-care workers. People who had been paying to not have to think about how certain kinds of work was getting done now needed to know: Does the person who cooked this meal for me have paid sick leave? Who cleans my office when I go home at night, and do they have enough time to do a reasonable job? How does my babysitter get to work? Who does my house cleaner live with?

People staying home looked around their houses and saw the need for care everywhere. To come alive to the centrality of care in this world is like waking up. The bed you lie in was designed and built by human hands, delivered and assembled by human hands. The sheet was fitted just so over the mattress by you, someone you love, or at least someone you trust enough to let into your bedroom.

"We are caught in an inescapable network of mutuality, tied in a single garment of destiny," wrote the Rev. Martin Luther King Jr. from Birmingham's jail.

And that garment is the cloth that someone swaddled you in when you were born, and it's also the shroud someone will pull over you when you die.

The force that connects us all is a constantly renewed choreography of care. Ai-Jen Poo, who devotes herself to lifting up domestic workers with the National Domestic Workers Alliance, says care is the work that makes other work possible.

The feminist economist Silvia Federici, originator of "wages for housework" campaigns in the 1970s, defines care as reproductive labor. This is a pun: it's both the labor that makes people and the kind that needs to be redone every day because it disappears without a trace—Sisyphus, doing the dishes.

Joan Tronto, a political scientist, is the author of the book *Caring Democracy* and a major theorist of care. She told me we need to flip the script of all our economics and our politics too.

We are encouraged to think of care for the young, old, and vulnerable as a humdrum activity that enables the productive work of the marketplace and the adult realm of politics. Instead, consider that the purpose of the economy is to support human flourishing. Therefore, the things we do at our "jobs" are meaningful only inasmuch as they enable the necessary functions of care. And democracy is in fact the process for determining the proper allocation of caring responsibilities.

The market is unable to account for either the cost or the value of care. If you were to "cost it out," it would be entirely unaffordable. The market wages of a full-time stay-at-home parent, with all the services they provide, from cleaning to cooking to organizing and planning and entertaining and educating, would be some $180,000 a year. Therefore, Tronto writes, our economic order rests on the ideological assertion that care is "natural."

Caring, a natural resource, like water or trees—neglected, overexploited, endangered, like water or trees.

Nancy Folbre, another feminist economist, in her masterwork *The Invisible Heart*, says care is systematically devalued exactly because it is priceless. We want the person who cares to *really care*. Emotional labor is part of the work. We don't want people who are in it for the money.

A wrenching scene illustrating Folbre's point comes from Miranda July's 2020 movie *Kajillionaire*. It's about a family of cold, craven, sociopathic grifters. At the climax, the grown daughter suddenly realizes the perversity of how she was raised. She challenges her mother to call her "hon."

"You can't do it. I bet you could if it was a job, though, right?" And she brandishes a check at her mother. "$1,575 to call me hon."

It's not possible to pay for care in this way. You can't slip Berg twenty dollars to hug your baby more warmly.

But we also can't afford anymore not to care for the people who care for us. And that includes making sure they have enough money to live with dignity.

By August 2021, employment across the economy had rebounded to 92 percent of pre-pandemic levels. But childcare had only bounced back to 88 percent, with 126,000 open positions. Wages were still abysmal, and caregivers could easily find fast-food or retail jobs that paid more.

In January 2021, Tronto told me she was optimistic. "I think we're at a moment when some of that is cracking open. People see the injustice of the way we've organized society. The question—the real question for me—is whether or not we have the wherewithal to pull that all together and say there's a different way to organize society."

CHILDREN PLAY THE PANDEMIC

Through all the trials of the past year, caregivers like Berg found their solace where they always had: in the children. "The kind of hope, or miracle story, is the children themselves, because they are so resilient. They just, they take change better than adults do. They still play. They still talk."

Children were demanding masks for their stuffed bears and baby dolls to wear. At one school, Berg saw "the kids had taken a little play plastic hair dryer, and they were using it like it was a [forehead] thermometer, taking temperatures of each other. You know, as soon as you start seeing children play their lived experience, that's a good sign."

Kathryn May, an emergency room nurse, had a toddler daughter in Berg's school when COVID hit. She said that through their face masks and their shields, the staff was able to project warmth with their voices and make the school feel safe and welcoming. "It was amazing because I didn't have the stress of 'where my child's going to go, who's going to watch my kid while I'm working? Who's going to be making sure everything is OK there? How is my husband going to be able to work if I'm at work?' Because if we didn't have that for her, then there were many days that I wasn't able to go to work because there was nobody to watch her."

May said that Berg's childcare center did a better, more consistent job providing care and communicating their plans than the Dallas public schools, where her older son was enrolled, and which opened full-time in the fall. "All of those systems that she's been so detailed about and focused on have allowed the school to be open this entire time. . . . Having that consistency and not having to be concerned that because there's a failure in the protocols or the systems that are set up, that we aren't going to have a lapse in coverage—that really just gives you a peace of mind and an ease."

HELP IS COMING

Eventually, Biden, like lots of other grandpas all around the country, decided to help out. Relief to the industry reached $50 billion through the spring of 2021. There was also relief extended directly to parents in his first package: a universal child cash benefit and an increase in the existing childcare tax credit.

Biden planned for more. The American Families Plan included $225 billion in childcare subsidies aimed at both sides of the otherwise unworkable care equation: to limit the costs to families and also raise wages for workers. Plus, $200 billion to give all three- and four-year-olds access to free public preschool.

SAFETY QUESTIONS AND DATA VOIDS

But what about the many, many children in families like Heather's, who didn't have that weight taken off their shoulders? Those whose childcare arrangements fell apart when COVID hit, who had no backup plan?

It's hard to know exactly how many children, like Heather's son Habersham, might have come to harm specifically because of gaps in supervision. In April, at the height of lockdown, only half of workers told Gallup they were fully remote, so clearly there were many children at home with fewer adults on hand.

One study found a significant rise in gun injuries among children under twelve, like Habersham, during the first six months of the pandemic, compared to the average for the few years before. Children also fired more guns on others: 106 times, causing forty-four deaths, compared to 71 times the year before. Guns are far more likely to be present in family homes than in schools or licensed childcare centers. Calls to poison control hotlines also spiked by about 70 percent year over year in the first several months of the pandemic.

Overall, though, fewer children were brought to emergency rooms in the early phase of the pandemic, as parents understandably avoided overwhelmed hospitals. The major sources of accidents and injury—sports and playgrounds—were shut down. Children were also taking fewer car trips; motor vehicle accidents are the leading cause of death for children five through fourteen.

The bottom line is, we don't have comprehensive evidence either way. Children were physically safer at home in some ways, in more physical danger in other ways. Children whose grownups were busy with work, stressed with economic troubles, and concerned about the pandemic itself felt lonely and neglected, angry and alienated, anxious and overwhelmed. These children suffered setbacks in their mental health, social development, and in many cases their education.

But what is also a compelling and pervasive reality is that parents and other caregivers stretched themselves to the limit and beyond to keep children safe when every other institution failed them. They did what they always did: they cared.

4 SPECIAL EDUCATION

We will be today terminating our relationship with the World Health Organization.

—Trump, May 29, 2020

May 27, 2020, US death toll passes 100,000

A small blue house on a steep street in San Francisco. Eleven-year-old Jonah is up by 6:00 a.m. But he refuses to get out of bed, his overgrown brown curls peeking from under the blankets. His mother, Maya, offers him a muffin from Philz Coffee; he won't eat. She puts him in front of the computer for the start of school.

Jonah's behavioral therapists had been unreliable since lockdown started—they'd cycled through five different people on his team in just four weeks. His moods were at their worst. He was severely opposed to Zoom school.

"Zoom just sucks," he told me. "It makes me extremely bored and anxious. You don't really learn anything on Zoom. I miss friends, having recess. We'd have these giant games of tag. We'd play army tag, with like twenty people from all the different grades, the whole recess."

If left alone for a minute, he'll switch to YouTube or a video game. He's become skilled at breaking whatever security they try to put on the computer. So Maya or Robert have to sit nearby at the dining table. They try to keep him on task by rewarding him with a piece of candy for every fifteen minutes he stays in his Zoom classroom with the camera on. "Sugar is a major food group in our house," Maya says.

Today, it's hopeless. The teacher squanders eight of those precious fifteen minutes taking roll. When she eventually gets around to asking the class a question, Maya prompts Jonah to participate. Jonah slams the computer against the table, breaking it for the third time since school went virtual.

Meanwhile, Maya and Robert both have work calls. And Maya needs to join her mother's doctor's visit by Zoom for the results of her lung scan.

Maya tries to get the broken computer away from Jonah. He grabs her phone and throws it to the ground. He kicks Robert in the crotch and yells at both of them. "I hate you! You're ugly! You're fat! I want to die. I wish I could kill myself. I want you to kill me!"

Maya is flooded with rage. She freely admits that her temper can match her son's at times, and quarantine seems to bring out the worst in everybody on a daily basis. Jonah starts crying and runs upstairs. He says he's not going to do school the rest of the day.

Maya is exhausted. The day is shot. It's barely nine in the morning.

WHAT LOST SCHOOLING MEANT FOR CHILDREN WITH DISABILITIES

This chapter tells the stories of Jonah and Alexis, 2 of the 7.3 million children, aged three through twenty-one, who receive federally subsidized services through the Individuals with Disabilities Education Act.

Each of these children is just that, an individual. Special education includes those with a specific learning disability such as dyslexia or auditory processing disorder; speech, visual, or hearing impairments; health issues like epilepsy or Tourette's syndrome or chronic illnesses that make it hard for them to sit through a regular school day; autism; mental health conditions that interfere with their learning such as obsessive-compulsive disorder (OCD) or anxiety; and various combinations of any of the above.

Children in special education had a vast range of experiences during the pandemic.

There were a few families who told me their children did better with remote learning than they did in the classroom. They may have had a home that was comfortable and a caring adult in the room who was able to provide continuous one-to-one support. Maybe the technology allowed them certain accommodations that weren't easy to do in the classroom. Dara Kass's middle son, Charlie, who has ADHD, felt like he was living his "best life" going to school from home and working at his own pace.

In many, many other cases, however, children with disabilities did much worse without in-person learning and therapies. They didn't just miss learning that could be made up later. They regressed in ways that might, in some cases, be permanent. Developmental disabilities follow developmental pathways, which is why there's so much emphasis on early intervention for these kids. Time is of the essence, and that's exactly what these children lost.

JONAH HAD A PLAN THAT WAS WORKING

Jonah's mom, Maya, had him on her own. Maya was in her thirties at the time, a queer food security activist in the Bay Area. She had a full life and thought of herself as too much of a "freak" to have children. But she gave herself a year to consider it, reading books and interviewing some nontraditional families she knew. "Eventually I decided that I would regret if I didn't do it," she told me. She decided to become a single mother by choice. By the age of thirty-eight she was pregnant.

Her baby boy was magnetic, with a quick sense of humor, curls, and freckles. He could also be explosive and destructive. Jonah's preschool teachers were the first to help Maya realize that he needed special intervention and support.

For years, Maya worked the system to get her son the proper evaluations and services. She had taken a job at a nonprofit, so she knew San Francisco's community-based organizations well. She was utterly determined advocating on behalf of her son. She knew some people thought she was hard to work with, but she didn't care as long as they did their jobs. She accepted a diagnosis of autism for Jonah because of the publicly funded interventions that came with it, although experts agreed Jonah was borderline; he was verbal, socially engaged, and affectionate with his mom and others. There could be daily "I hate yous" but also daily "I love yous."

By the spring of fifth grade, after years of phone calls, meetings, lobbying, and paperwork, Jonah was getting support for his dyslexia in small groups during the school day. A behavioral therapist was coming to the house almost every day and established a reward system for the smallest positive responses, in a sometimes controversial therapy for autism called applied behavioral analysis. Then everything shut down, and their daily life became an exhausting battle.

ALEXIS MISSES HER CLASSMATES

Vanessa Ince's daughter, Alexis, has blonde pigtails and glasses. She also has a rare chromosomal abnormality and autism. When she started at her elementary school in Maui, Hawaii, at the age of eight, in 2018, she was the size of a three-year-old and was nonverbal.

Vanessa worried she'd be bullied. But Alexis thrived at school. Her peers surrounded her with kindness, taking turns guiding her through her day. Because she couldn't greet them with words, the teachers arranged for her to put a lei of flowers around her friends' necks each morning, in the traditional Hawaiian gesture of welcome.

Then the pandemic closed schools. And Alexis, now age ten, couldn't understand why. Vanessa called it "devastating."

She seemed to be pining for her friends, her routines, the structure and the stimulation of school. She went from a "happy, bubbly, loving-life child" to "flat and empty and not really there. Like a robot." She wouldn't sit still for more than fifteen seconds; she wandered their house as though she were looking for her friends. To Vanessa, who is a psychologist, it seemed as if her daughter had the classic symptoms of depression, though it's hard for her to tell her family how she is feeling.

Alexis also regressed, a sign of severe stress in children. She went back from being almost completely potty trained to needing diapers. She went back to crawling instead of walking, and stopped trying to use her communication device.

This regression was heartbreaking. And it meant Alexis's education plan, based on her previous evaluation in February 2020, was no longer relevant. Vanessa and her husband filed a lawsuit seeking to get Hawaii's Department of Education to pay for the services Alexis needs in a facility where she could see other children.

SPECIAL EDUCATION IS AN ADVERSARIAL SYSTEM

It may seem extreme that Alexis's family considered it necessary to file a lawsuit in the middle of a pandemic to get her what she needed. But it's actually pretty common in the adversarial world of special education.

The formal education of children with disabilities dates to the early nineteenth century. Similar to the day nursery movement around the same time, these early efforts tended to be private experiments founded by upper-class philanthropists with a scientific curiosity about various conditions.

Thomas Hopkins Gallaudet, whose background was as a minister and a traveling salesman, established the American School for the Deaf in Hartford, Connecticut, in 1817. It was distinguished from similar institutions in Europe for teaching sign language rather than lipreading. The first US institutions for the blind were opened in Boston, New York, and Philadelphia in 1832 and 1833.

Some of these institutions branched out to educate people with intellectual disabilities. Dr. Samuel Gridley Howe, director of the Perkins School for the Blind, established the first such dedicated school in 1848 in South Boston, with a name that gives a glimpse at how these human beings were seen at the time: the Massachusetts School for Idiotic and Feeble-Minded Youth.

In the late nineteenth century, rising immigration, compulsory attendance, and child labor laws massively increased school enrollment. Schools no longer had the privilege of educating only those students whose parents were most determined that they get an education or those who most wanted to be there. The result was wholly predictable: as schools took in a wider range of children, they found more of them failed to pass through the narrow portal that had been shaped for a lucky few.

Ellwood Cubberley, a historian of education and a major force in teacher education at Stanford University, wrote in 1912 that schools, as he saw it, were increasingly burdened with a long list of undesirables. To wit: "the truant," "the incorrigible," "the sick, needy, and physically unfit," the "crippled, tubercular, deaf, epileptic, and blind," "many children of the foreign-born who have no aptitude for book learning," and "many children of inferior mental qualities."

Around this time, IQ tests arose as a supposedly scientific method of screening for such "defectives." Almost two million World War I recruits took a version of these tests, with about half scoring at a mental age of below twelve years old.

Early IQ proponents like Lewis Terman and Henry Goddard were anti-immigrant and eugenicist. Terman, who helped adapt the tests for US use, suggested that there were "enormously significant racial differences in general intelligence." Rather, enduring racism in society affects both how we conceive of and how we measure intelligence.

By the 1920s, using standardized tests adapted from the IQ model, millions of US students were sorted and ranked on a bell curve each year, with approximately 14 percent declared "accelerated" and 15 percent "retarded." It may or may not be a coincidence that almost the same proportion of schoolchildren today, about 14 percent nationwide, are classified as needing special education services.

Schools responded largely by segregating the students who didn't move at the same pace as everyone else and offering them less. States passed laws providing exceptions to the rule of compulsory attendance, which allowed public schools to refuse to admit children deemed unable to benefit from the education offered there.

Many such young people were shunted to overage, ungraded classes, given trades or crafts instead of academics, or most ominously, sent away to state "industrial" or "reform" schools and asylums, which warehoused about fifty thousand boys and twelve thousand girls nationwide by 1910, according to Cubberley.

WILLOWBROOK: THE LAST GREAT DISGRACE

Institutional abuse of intellectually disabled children continued for decades. A 1972 television exposé by a young Geraldo Rivera brought national attention to the horrors at a state institution for mentally disabled children and adults, Willowbrook Hospital, in Staten Island. Children were being beaten, starved, tied up in straitjackets, and neglected in filthy conditions that Senator Robert F. Kennedy had called "a snake pit" several years earlier, in a 1965 visit to the facility. (Kennedy's own sister Rosemary, who had developmental disabilities, was institutionalized after a lobotomy.)

On behalf of residents and their parents, the New York Civil Liberties Union and the Legal Aid Society filed class action lawsuits over the conditions at Willowbrook. The eventual consent judgment in 1973 stopped short of affirming a constitutional right to education for these children. But it did recognize that they, "regardless of the degree of handicapping conditions, are capable of physical, intellectual, emotional and social growth, and...a certain level of affirmative intervention and programming is necessary if that capacity for growth and development is to be preserved, and regression prevented."

THE FIGHT FOR EQUAL ACCESS

The fight for inclusion for students with disabilities, not to mention the recognition of their full humanity, grew directly out of the struggle for racial justice. *Brown v. Board of Education*, the 1954 Supreme Court decision, with its guarantees of equal access to education for all, became the legal basis for special education rights.

A series of court decisions in the 1960s and 1970s established an adversarial, legalistic dynamic in the special education world: children could not be excluded from school without due process and a fair hearing to determine the best setting for their needs. Parents of special education students were thrust into the role of advocates. Their children wouldn't be guaranteed access to school unless they fought for it, one by one.

The "free, appropriate public education" guaranteed by the Individuals with Disabilities Education Act must be provided in the "least restrictive environment." This means, to the extent possible, students should be attending regular schools, in regular classrooms, with their peers.

The accommodations children in special education need to thrive can range from a little extra time on tests, to a personal aide assigned to them all day long, to full-time placement in a residential program.

But one thing is true: special ed costs more than general ed—twice as much or more, on average. Money spent on special education comes out of school budgets, and public school districts are always short on cash. The federal government picks up only a fraction of the tab for special ed. That means getting schools to live up to the law takes an enormous amount of time and energy.

NOTHING WITHOUT A STRUGGLE

There is one particular type of person who does the vast majority of research, advocacy, and direct support of a child with disabilities. That is usually their mother. These mothers leave the workforce in large numbers. Their marriages break down more often, and their mental health suffers. That's all true even when there's not a pandemic.

Specialized lawyers, advocates, and private evaluators have cropped up to help families overcome a complex and sometimes obstructionist bureaucracy to first have their children identified for services and then to actually get them the services they're entitled to. It takes money, education, and other forms of social capital to navigate this system.

"Nothing about the educational guarantees and provisions of service that we have today for all students with disabilities came without a struggle," observes Wanda Blanchett, a special education scholar at Rutgers University. "Never yet have we achieved in this country those guarantees for all children."

As has been true for generations, disability rights and other civil rights continue to intersect. Children of color and those growing up in poverty are more likely—some scholars, like Blanchett, say too likely—to be classified as needing special education, based on their test scores and other indicators. At the same time, they are less likely to get appropriate services in the most inclusive settings. So special education in practice, Blanchett and other scholars argue, is a form of legalized segregation.

MOST CHILDREN IN SPECIAL EDUCATION DID WORSE DURING COVID

There were silver linings to the transition to online learning, at least for a lucky few.

Students who used wheelchairs or were chronically ill no longer had to exhaust themselves moving from classroom to classroom or waiting for the elevator in less accessible buildings. With the right support at home, children with hearing loss could watch their teachers' video lectures with closed captioning. If they had trouble focusing, they could pause and rewatch. If they had a stutter or social anxiety and didn't like to speak up in class, now they could ask questions over chat.

In my own daughter's private Montessori classroom, there was a little boy who had been diagnosed with non-Hodgkin's lymphoma in December 2019. When the class switched to Zoom circle time in March 2020, he and his friends were reunited, each in their own home.

But most children who struggled with learning in any way, whether designated special ed or not, were not getting what they needed over a computer screen. In a national survey conducted in May 2020, only one in five parents reported their children in special education were receiving all the services they were entitled to. Twice as many, 39 percent, of parents reported their children were not receiving any services at all.

Some families, like Alexis's and Jonah's, had private insurance that could pay for in-person services. Many did not.

The toll was not only academic or developmental. That same survey found four in ten parents of children in special education were concerned about their children's mental health, almost twice the proportion of parents whose children were not in special education.

SPINS AND FALLS

Jonah's one true love, besides technology, is his Razor scooter. For months the skate parks were closed. "We went to this one place in Daly City—it was closed because of COVID. And it wasn't just like closed, they were like NOOO SKATERS!!! And they put chains all the way THROUGH the park. It was like a laser maze or something." But by summer 2020 they were starting to open again, and Maya and Robert drove him to pretty much every skate park in the Bay Area.

Jonah seems to find a different kind of focus when he's nailing tricks on his scooter. "A Taylor spin is—so the bottom of the scooter, you make it do a 360. You jump, you spin, and you land. I can do two of them in a row. I landed my first one [in July 2020], it was pretty sloppy but I landed it." He also asks his parents to film pretty much every run. He edits the clips and rewatches them endlessly or replays them for anyone who will sit still.

At the end of August, Maya found a spot for him in day camp. She was eager, bordering on desperate, to get him out of the house, but he didn't know anyone, and the small pod they had placed him with was all girls, which was hard for him socially. Jonah started refusing to go, and he put all his considerable will into that refusal. One morning, a Monday about two weeks before school started, Maya had him at the gate of the camp.

"I was trying to get him to not run away, like physically run out of the camp, so I could leave. And I think I had him by his backpack, and he literally swung me around and I fell on the ground." She remembers being sprawled out, sliding on the sidewalk, in front of the staff. "And they were like, this isn't going to work. You can't leave him here." Maya hung her head.

"I picked Jonah up. I picked myself up. His eyes were huge. Then we just got in the car, and he's like, 'Sorry, Mom.' Oh my God. It was so mortifying and so sad. We just had to sit there for a minute."

SUITS FILED

Starting in the spring of 2020, parents of students in special education sued and filed complaints against schools and state education departments, various states, districts, the US Department of Education, and the Bureau of Indian Education over the denial of special education services required by law.

The Inces' attorney, Keith Peck, filed a suit seeking class action status that covered all families in the state whose children's individualized education plans were breached during the pandemic. A federal class action suit was filed in July 2020 on the same grounds.

These suits generally ask for damages that include extra time and extra teaching and therapy. That's a concept in special education law known as "compensatory services."

All this legal action was, unfortunately, unlikely to deliver swift or satisfying relief. For one thing, education departments could claim force majeure—that an "act of God" stopped them from doing their jobs.

And the adversarial process of redressing individual complaints threatened to overwhelm already-weakened school systems. It's entirely possible that when all is said and done, districts and states end up spending more money fighting families in court over COVID-related denial of services, and on paying families' legal fees when they lose, than they spend on the services themselves. Meanwhile, months become years and children grow up.

There's yet another practical problem: teachers and other specialists were overwhelmed and burned out several months into the pandemic. Special education direct service providers are mostly women. Many of these practitioners were raising children of their own and under their own impossible stress. In many places there isn't a ready pipeline of new providers for all the extra services children may need in the months and years to come.

Blanchett found herself most concerned about the families who might have lost services because of COVID yet didn't have the wherewithal to be the squeaky wheel. "It's certainly highly likely that some of the kids that need the most services are not receiving them. And they will have the most dire consequences. If your parents don't have the means to supplement services that aren't being provided by school districts, we're going to see even more regression there."

FEWER BABIES GETTING HELP

In recent years publicly funded early intervention for infants to three-year-olds has grown. The sooner something like a speech or motor delay can be identified and treated, the better the outcomes tend to be. But during 2020, referrals dropped, and so did the rate of services provided. Babies were missing routine checkups, toddlers weren't going to daycare, and there was no one from outside the home who could flag missed milestones. This lapse in services to the youngest children could reverberate for the next two decades.

Patricia, in DC, had professional training in special education and still dealt with a dearth of services for PJ that may have delayed his learning to walk and talk. In the fall of 2020, a doctor told Heather, in St. Louis, that her baby daughter, Shekitha, appeared to have autism. Since she couldn't find any open daycare to send any of her children to, it didn't seem realistic to her to try to find special therapists.

EXCRUCIATING CHOICES

As schools started in the fall of 2020, some families, like Alexis's, wanted in-person learning. Yet federal data released for the first time during the Biden administration suggested they wouldn't get to the head of the line. A minority, four in ten districts, even claimed to be giving priority to students with disabilities for in-person instruction in the spring of 2021. In practice, students with disabilities were, if anything, a little more likely to remain remote.

I heard from some special education teachers that they worried their students would not be able to wear masks or wash their hands correctly. And they worried about transmission for those students who need help eating and help with the bathroom.

Hawaii did bring special education students back to school. But it was an excruciating choice. Alexis is in delicate health and uses a feeding tube. Vanessa was terrified of her getting COVID-19. "Do we keep her home, you know, in a bubble or do we send her out into the world and risk her getting something that can kill her?" Ultimately, she concluded that she had to take the risk. "She had just shut down so much of her life. She's barely even here. She's a shell of a child."

School with COVID protocols in place didn't bring all the benefits Vanessa had hoped for. Alexis apparently had trouble hearing and understanding her teachers through the masks and face shields. She wasn't able to interact with other special education students because of social distancing. The general education classmates who had embraced her so warmly weren't there anymore. "She would just stand on the curb in the morning when I took her to school, just looking confused. And just kind of wandering around. It was heartbreaking."

By the spring of 2021, the family's lawsuit had progressed to an appeal. School, which used to be a haven for Alexis, had become a place where Vanessa felt singled out as a troublemaker for trying to advocate for her child. Alexis was still in diapers, still downcast, and still, in Vanessa's opinion, not receiving the services she needed.

"I feel so outraged," Vanessa told me. "It's just so unjust. And honestly, [I'm] perplexed and confused. I don't understand why the Department of Education does this. It makes no sense. It's very clear, even to a layperson, what this child needs. It's hard to wrap your mind around that kind of nonsensical behavior, cruel behavior."

Vanessa and her husband tried hard to make up for everything Alexis wasn't getting at school. They had the advanced degrees, the extra money, and the time to do it. And they saw some gains. "We hire people to work with Alexis at home. We spend much more, like, devoted one-on-one attention, directed attention…trying to teach her things instead of just being able to have fun and play with her. We have very little time to try [to] get her back on track. So we're trying to be a little bit more focused and structured in our interactions with her. So she's actually learning more."

LIFE WITHOUT A LOT OF OTHER OPTIONS

In the fall of 2020, if possible, things get worse for Jonah and Maya. It's sixth grade. Jonah has to start remotely at a new school where he doesn't know any of the teachers. He finds virtual class unbearably boring.

There are more physical attacks, more thrown and broken electronics. He will rip the cord of Maya's computer out of the wall while she is trying to work in a corner of the crowded living room.

Although they all fantasize about severing from the hell that is Zoom school, Jonah doesn't have a lot of other options. As exhausting as it is already to manage virtual school, Maya can't contemplate homeschooling him. She doesn't have the mental strength or patience to fill all of his hours herself. She's not financially able to leave her job to do it. While there are very expensive private schools that specialize in serving students with needs like Jonah's, a lot of special education families find that generalized private schools aren't willing or able to accommodate them, especially a kid with Jonah's behaviors.

San Francisco's public schools stay all virtual well into the spring. But the city, like others around the country, opens "learning hubs" in locations like recreation centers, libraries, and some school buildings. They are intended for the city's most vulnerable students and those whose parents are essential workers.

Maya snags Jonah a spot at one. She is relieved by the prospect of some much-needed peace and quiet for a few hours during the day. Then it didn't work out; it was a long drive in morning traffic, and Jonah got in trouble constantly. She said the staff wasn't willing or able to follow Jonah's behavior plan.

On good days Maya tries to get Jonah out of the house for a walk before school starts—the more physical activity, the better. One of the few bright spots in his days is their extremely patient black-and-white cat, Teddy. "We call him the emotional support cat," Jonah says. "He is very cute, very nice, and very fluffy."

On the fridge is a list of things that Jonah can do instead of cursing or hitting or throwing things when he gets mad and out of control: deep breathing or cuddling Teddy or lying like a starfish spread out on the bed. And a list of reward activities; electronics are still his major motivator.

Jonah has lost all interest in reading or writing. He doesn't seem to have absorbed much math or science, except for the physics required to do a 1080—a triple rotation—on his scooter. Sometimes, he seemed not only full of rage but hopeless and joyless. Nothing is fun or interesting anymore.

But his family keeps trying. Every night they eat dinner at six, usually plain chicken or something else simple. Jonah's in bed by 8:00 p.m. He's always been a good sleeper. His mother reads to him, often from a book of essays for adults called *Seeing Nature: Deliberate Encounters with the Visible World*. It's an extended and complex meditation on energy flows and change, for example how water cuts rock deep into a canyon.

Bedtime is also the best time for apologies and repair. "I do feel that one thing that we've gotten really much better at during this pandemic is apologizing and starting over," Maya says. "I know I say things I shouldn't, but I'm good at kind of letting things go. [And] I think Jonah's really gotten better at it, too, taking my apology."

WHAT SPECIAL EDUCATION HAS TO TELL US

A lot of parents can probably relate to how Jonah's days blurred together in a dense grid of schedules, behavior charts, and plans that got crumpled up and replaced with other plans. Not to mention how Maya completely lost her patience and somehow survived to do it all over again the next day. I know I can.

I've heard it said that most public education should work like special education does—when it is actually working. Don't all children deserve an individualized plan that takes into account their strengths, weaknesses, and particular goals? Wouldn't it be ideal for teachers to get a behavior plan outlining the kinds of incentives and consequences your child is most likely to respond to?

This idea might be especially true after the pandemic, when uneven access to school left our kids in such different places developmentally, academically, and socially.

But the outright denial of services to so many, the adversarial system that drains everyone's energy scrapping for scarce resources, and the toll on mothers in particular don't sound like much of a model for the rest of the education system to follow.

We'll hear from Jonah's family again in Chapter 6; things get even more complicated for them but also a little less lonely for Jonah.

SUMMER 2020

5   RACISM

These THUGS are dishonoring the memory of George Floyd, and I won't let that happen. Just spoke to Governor Tim Walz and told him that the Military is with him all the way. Any difficulty and we will assume control but, when the looting starts, the shooting starts. Thank you!

—President Trump, via Twitter, May 29, 2020

June 1, 2020, US seven-day average of cases: 21,518

By May, Patricia Stamper's toddler, Patrick, seemed increasingly uncomfortable. He would whimper and pull at his diaper. He still wasn't walking, though he was closer to two years old than one. He would stand holding on to furniture in the family's half of a duplex in Deanwood, their historic, predominantly Black Washington, DC, neighborhood.

Patricia and Pete were concerned enough to take him to the doctor. They determined he had an inguinal hernia, a symptom of his genetic disorder. He would need surgery.

While they were dealing with this news, the neighborhood, the city, and the country exploded around them. On May 25, a white Minneapolis police officer named Derek Chauvin murdered a forty-six-year-old Black man named George Floyd in broad daylight on a public street.

Darnella Frazier, a seventeen-year-old girl who was out that day buying her nine-year-old cousin a snack, recorded the murder with her cell phone and posted it to social media. The video, which showed Floyd pleading for his life, spread like a grass fire. Frazier would go on to win a special Pulitzer citation for her act of witness.

TO THE STREETS

Americans who had been living under lockdown, avoiding public gatherings, swarmed the streets in protest. So did people from Guam to Reykjavik.

By some estimates, this was the largest street protest movement in US history. Polls suggested as many as twenty-six million Americans turned out in total; half a million on a single day, June 6.

The media dwelled on the most frightening images: a police vehicle on fire, cops in riot gear. But the demonstrations, marches, and vigils were almost entirely peaceful. An analysis of more than seventy-three hundred of these events showed protesters or bystanders were reported injured in just 1.6 percent of the events, and police far less often. Police gassed protestors 2.5 percent of the time.

Patricia was angry and sad about George Floyd, and about the intensity of police response to the protesters, and about a lifetime of living with racism. "When we march, you're mad. When we kneel, you're mad. When we protest peacefully, you're mad. When we sit at your lunch counters, you're mad. When we go to church! So what do you want me to do, go home? No. You kidnapped my ancestors, but now I'm here. I got no home to go to."

This was a youth-led movement, starting with Darnella Frazier. Many protests were organized by high school students, and not only those who were Black. Like sixteen-year-old Ayesha Chaudhry, who organized a Black Lives Matter march in Mason, Ohio, her largely Republican Cincinnati suburb, with a multiracial group of girlfriends who met in their AP Government class. The peaceful demonstration stretched four blocks long.

Chaudhry immigrated from Pakistan as a child; English is her second language. In her spare time she posts makeup tutorials to Instagram. One day she dreams of being an attorney for the ACLU. "I think that's one thing that definitely gets misconstrued [about teenagers], is that we're ungrateful. And I'm not ungrateful," she told me. "I'm so, so, so grateful for the life that America has provided me. But it's because I'm so grateful for that life that I'm willing to fight for America and willing to fight for American citizens' liberties, and making sure that they're living in a place that they love."

TEENAGE WASTELAND

For teens like Chaudhry, getting out in the street was more than a political exercise. It was catharsis, after a season of monotony and confinement. The remote half semester was crawling to an end. Few school buildings had reopened across the country, with the exception of some tiny rural districts in places like Wyoming and Montana. Some districts had ended the school year early, in exhaustion or defeat. High school graduates were giving valedictory addresses over Zoom, posing for faux "prom" photos without the actual dance, picking up diplomas by car parade.

Nationally, seniors graduated at about the same rate as previous years—often because high schools ignored their performance after school went remote. And the pandemic accelerated a preexisting trend of colleges no longer requiring applicants to submit ACT or SAT scores. A total of two-thirds of all degree-granting institutions nationwide dropped their test requirements. Nevertheless, the fall of 2020 saw an unprecedented 13 percent drop in the number of students entering college for the first time. This decline was led by community colleges, suggesting that working-class students in particular were at risk of falling off the college track for good, just as studies of past disasters would predict.

CANCEL CAMP

Children were facing a bleak summer. Camps and programs like the Fresh Air Fund were canceled or cut back. City-sponsored youth employment programs were cut in New York, and went virtual or partly virtual in DC and Los Angeles. Cities like New York were finally reopening playgrounds that had been padlocked for months, but not their public pools. Los Angeles kept its playgrounds shut through October 2020, despite mounting evidence that COVID did not easily transmit outdoors.

The lack of organized and outdoor play for children would take a toll on their health. A large national study found that children gained weight twice as fast from March to November 2020 as in similar time periods pre-pandemic.

They may have turned to emotional eating because they were bored or depressed. Patricia Stamper in DC, working as a special education classroom aide, recalled watching one of her students gain weight steadily over Zoom. "He was home with his grandmother. Every time he was on camera, he was eating." Two studies conducted at two different hospitals each found a doubling in the number of children hospitalized for diabetes in March 2020–March 2021 compared to the year before. The overall numbers in these studies were small, in the double digits. It may be that more of these children showed up sick enough to be admitted to the hospital because their parents had waited too long to bring them in for treatment due to COVID fears. Still, without concerted effort and intervention, it's fair to assume more children risk lifelong health problems because of this period of enforced inactivity.

Dr. Dara Kass published an op-ed in the *New York Times* on May 27 headlined, "Cancel Sleepaway Camp." She had been a camp doctor and started a company offering medical advice to camps, so the piece didn't make her any friends, least of all among her children. "We know this isn't easy to hear," Dara and her coauthor wrote. "This is yet another loss in the coronavirus era. As parents and doctors we understand this deeply."

About two out of three camps, particularly overnight camps, stayed closed for the summer of 2020. And those that opened had outbreaks, including one at a maskless camp in Georgia where more than four in ten staff and campers got the virus.

Dara made the call in the name of equity and priorities. Testing capacity still wasn't where it needed to be, and rather than use coronavirus tests for camps, she thought authorities should focus on schools. "We had to invest in schools if we ever wanted them open," she told me. She was hoping that frequent and rapid testing could allow schools to stay open. In the end few public schools, still, were given the resources to do that in the fall of 2020.

"There is an adage in medicine: 'We don't always have to be right, but we can't afford to be wrong,'" read the op-ed. "This is especially true for a disease whose effect on children is just now coming into view." They were referring to emerging cases of multisystem inflammatory syndrome, a complication that could turn up in children four or more weeks after a COVID infection. The CDC started tracking cases in mid-May 2020. The scary and mysterious syndrome gained plenty of media coverage. But despite early fears, it remained rare. There were fewer than four thousand cases from May 2020 to May 2021, and 99 percent of patients recovered.

BACKGROUND NOISE

Cases had been falling since early April's peaks in hotspots, which included Detroit and New Orleans as well as New York City. Yet having lived through the peak in New York, Dara saw new waves starting to build elsewhere. "I'm looking at the national numbers and I can see kind of what I call background noise. Like a radio, I start hearing the static." Lockdowns were lifting, and there still wasn't sufficient testing, or tracing, or honest and consistent public messaging.

Nor were there, in most places, clear plans or public messages in place about a return to in-person school in the fall. This was bad news, because normally schools start planning in April for the upcoming school year. Decisions about staffing and budgeting and scheduling have to be made if things are going to go smoothly.

With little direct guidance at the national level, different groups were pulling in different directions. The American Federation of Teachers, the nation's second-largest teacher union, with its membership concentrated in New York State, put out a plan at the end of April that set out strict guidelines for reopening. Among other benchmarks, it called for two weeks of declining cases in a county before schools should even think about holding classes in person. In California, Governor Gavin Newsom made noises about opening up buildings for summer school as soon as July; he got swift pushback from district leaders, and the state's schools would ultimately remain closed longer than almost anywhere else.

While she was talking publicly about the summer, Dara was talking privately to schools about the fall. "I started advising a lot of the school systems on how to open. But I also knew that I could depend on nobody. I needed to figure out my own family's education." She was increasingly convinced that it would largely be up to individual parents to chart the path forward in the pandemic as best they could. And their success would be a function of privilege.

DAD, TEACHER, NURTURER OF BLACK LIVES

With COVID on the back burner for the moment, the isolation and hardship of the pandemic spring suddenly broke forth into a historic uprising for racial justice. I talked to Jesse Hagopian on June 2, 2020, while his home city of Seattle was under curfew in an attempt to control the protests. Hagopian is a father of two, a high school teacher, an author, and an activist, a founder of a national organization called Black Lives Matter at School. Their platform calls for Black history and ethnic studies, more teachers of color, equal funding, and the removal of police from schools.

Some of Hagopian's students at Garfield High School hadn't been logging in to class much that spring. They were sleeping on couches in doubled-up housing. They were working retail jobs to help support their families. And now they were out on the streets protesting. "Many of them are very active in the struggle that's going on right now. And I think they're getting a whole different education. I don't think their schooling is stopped at all. I think, if anything, it's on hyperdrive. They're learning a lot about how this world works and what it takes to create change. And those will be lessons they take with them for a long time."

He was proud of his students. But it was also a time of violence, fear of violence, and traumatic recollections of past violence for children of color. Not least for Hagopian's own two young sons.

On Saturday, May 30, 2020, Hagopian, his wife, and his sons, then seven and eleven, went to a rally. "And we were there for about twenty minutes listening to speeches and chants before the police shot a flashbang into the crowd, just seemingly unprovoked and out of nowhere. And then the smoke was rising. People were screaming. Everyone was running as fast as they can away. And my kids were really rattled and upset."

Especially his younger son, who still remembered a formative incident from several years before. Hagopian was speaking at a Martin Luther King Day rally when he was pepper-sprayed in the face by a police officer. It was the day of his son's second birthday party. "It was horrific pain. I got to his party late. I spent the party pouring milk in my eyes and my face and it was traumatizing to him. So he's been knowing what police violence is about for most of his life."

Hagopian filed a federal lawsuit against the police department. They settled for $100,000 without admitting guilt. All of it led to him having a version of what Black and Brown parents call "the talk"—telling their children how to keep safe and avoid the threat posed by police—much earlier than he wanted to. "I've had to have some very difficult talks that I wish I didn't have to have yet with my kids about this moment, and about police violence. And it's challenging because I don't want to have them paralyzed with fear and tell them some of the most gruesome, horrific details of what police are doing. At the same time, I need them to be safe and I need them to know that the police aren't always our friends."

Hagopian spent the weeks after George Floyd's death comforting both his students and his children. "He's learning from our experiences," he said of his younger son. "And what I try to do is give some context to it, help him process his emotions. And tell them he is not wrong for being scared, that it's nothing to be ashamed of. That it was OK to cry when we were at the rally. And I told him I would always keep him safe. So I'm just trying to hold them close right now."

MOTORCADE TO THE CATHEDRAL

Patricia's older boy, just five years old, was also frightened to tears by the police that same week of 2020. It wasn't at a march. She brought her sons to some Black Lives Matter gatherings a little later on in the summer that stayed peaceful.

But on June 1 the protests came to her.

Patricia put her two sons in their car seats that evening and headed for Children's National Medical Center, on Michigan Avenue, to get Patrick tested for COVID. He needed a negative result before his hernia surgery, which was scheduled for June 4.

She was stopped by the DC police. A motorcade was coming, they said.

"It was the day that Trump decided to go to the cathedral."

That very evening, police and National Guard troops used smoke, flash grenades, and tear gas to clear peaceful demonstrators from a public park, in what the *New York Times* called "a burst of violence unlike any seen in the shadow of the White House in generations." The violence was done on the order of Attorney General William Barr, so that President Trump could pose for photographs in front of the historic St. John's Episcopal Church, a short walk from the White House, holding a Bible.

That day he used words like "dominate," "vicious," "thugs," "law and order," as well as this threat: "I am dispatching thousands and thousands of heavily armed soldiers, military personnel and law enforcement officers to stop the rioting, looting, vandalism, assaults and the wanton destruction of property."

Trump's rhetoric traced back to his 2017 inaugural address, which had the action-movie-esque theme of "American carnage." The president and his allies must have seen a political advantage in stoking fear of violence and chaos. If necessary they were willing to create those conditions themselves.

SUMMONING ALL THE MAMAS

The Black Lives Matter movement in the summer of 2020 didn't soar on an updraft of violence and chaos. It rose on the energy of young people demanding a better world and the pain and strength of mothers. Among his last words, later witnessed around the world, George Floyd called out for his mother, dead two years: "Mama, mama, I'm through." One of the popular signs at the marches that followed read, "When George Floyd called out for his mama, he summoned all the mamas."

If you are a white reader of this book, let me say something to you, white person to white person: If you aspire to stand with all the mamas George Floyd summoned, it means reckoning in detail with how white supremacy is visited specifically on children. In lost jobs and household security. In laptops and textbooks. In death and loss.

But this chapter of the story is not just about oppression and victimhood. It's also about the unfinished fight for equality.

The other lost year.

And the new generation of freedom schools that rose up when the schoolhouse door was closed.

THE RACIAL TOLL OF COVID

For people of color in America, COVID-19 was a second pandemic on top of the preexisting pandemic of racism.

Asian Americans experienced a wave of hate crimes. President Trump repeatedly and publicly used language like "Chinese virus" and "kung flu" to describe the pandemic.

Latinx, Native American, and Black people were at greater risk than white or Asian Americans of being severely sickened and killed by COVID. They often died at far younger ages. This meant they more often left young children behind.

Latinx and, even more so, Black children were more likely than their white peers to get sicker from COVID. While multisystem inflammatory syndrome and other serious COVID complications were very rare in children, they were more common in children who weren't white.

There were several factors contributing to this. People of color were more likely to be working in low-wage "essential" occupations with more exposure to the virus, such as farming or retail. They also were more likely to be living in overcrowded and multigenerational households. And they were more likely to have conditions that made a COVID infection more dangerous, like diabetes or heart disease. These conditions can be attributed to the toll of racism, not genetics. They come from unequal exposure to what UK epidemiologist Michael Marmot calls the "social determinants of health," ranging from unsafe housing, to food deserts, to exposure to violence, stress, and trauma.

This in turn meant proportionately more Black and Brown children were bereaved by the pandemic.

REMEMBERING PAPI

In San Antonio, Texas, eleven-year-old Christian and fourteen-year-old Gisele Alfaro shared a bedroom with their papi, their mother's father. His snoring made them laugh.

"He was a really helpful person and really hardworking. He would make window screens for our neighbors. It just shines through in everything that he did," Christian told me. Papi woke his grandson up early on Saturdays for bike rides and attended his talent shows. Christian, who sports a mini-pompadour, is a self-taught musician whose repertoire includes "Bohemian Rhapsody" on the piano. Papi also made it to every one of Gisele's track meets and volleyball games.

On the Tuesday before Father's Day, in June, Papi started feeling sick. It took the family a few days to find a place where he could get tested. He went into the hospital, and the family had trouble getting updates from the nurses.

I remember praying a lot," said Christian. "My cousin, she would really help me. She would play some games with me, just keep me kind of busy and not worrying."

Gisele stayed busy with tasks around the house. "Of course I always worry, but I didn't want to worry as much because I thought that he was going to come home."

On July 14, his birthday, they managed to FaceTime him, but he was on a ventilator and unresponsive. Five days later he was gone. He was just fifty-seven years old. "We would spend a bunch of time together, and we had all these memories, but you can't make more," said Gisele.

Having more direct experience with death and severe illness from COVID changed how Black and Hispanic families viewed the dangers of the pandemic. In the fall, they would be generally more cautious, particularly less willing than white families to return to school in person.

Gisele and Christian stayed home throughout the 2020–2021 year, despite schools opening up in San Antonio. They were grieving and they were scared. "In the beginning, I thought this virus wasn't that serious. It was just like, stay away from people, stay home, wear masks. But now that we've lost a loved one, I felt like it put our whole family into a little panic," said Christian. "And, like, I think we developed anxiety to just go places."

Gisele skipped hanging out with her friends. In January she even canceled her own quinceañera, the blowout fifteenth birthday party that Latina girls look forward to throughout their childhoods. "It was kind of a hard decision, but also at the same time kind of easy. I just wanted to keep everyone safe and I didn't care about having a party anymore."

THE COST OF THE PANDEMIC

COVID's economic toll also fell harder on families of color. Four in ten Latina mothers and two-thirds of Black mothers are their families' breadwinners. These mothers were harder hit by job losses in sectors like food service, retail, and childcare. As of April 2020, they had higher unemployment rates than any other group—20 percent for Hispanic women and 17 percent for Black women, compared to 12 percent for white men.

Phil Fisher, at the University of Oregon, began surveying families with children under five at the very beginning of the pandemic. He found Black and Latinx households were much more likely to report material hardships, including problems paying for utilities and housing as well as food. The rate was 57 percent for Black families and 53 percent for Latinx families, compared to 40 percent overall.

Fisher also discovered that even if they earned a middle- or upper-middle-class income, families of color were less insulated from financial and material hardships than their white counterparts. There are several reasons why, he explained. "There's a wealth gap in households of color. So less savings and less ability to get credit. There's also a difference in the types of jobs. So even if people were earning enough to put them into the middle- or upper-income bracket, the jobs are less stable and more likely to go away. And also, Black and Latinx households are more likely to be paying to help support extended family members, even outside the household."

Patricia and Pete both kept their primary jobs during the pandemic, but money got tight. He was making Maryland's minimum wage, $11.75 an hour, as a caretaker on a golf course; his hours were reduced. Her job as a special education classroom aide for the DC public schools paid around $16 an hour. They went to the city for help paying the utility bills and rent. Just as Fisher described, Patricia and Pete also were surrounded by people even needier than they were. They contributed to fundraisers for health care, food, and home repairs for neighbors and family friends. "We put up money that we really didn't have, trying to help other people, you know, out of the kindness of your heart," as Patricia told me.

RACISM AND RESISTANCE

America's racial hierarchy is the engineered structure of the landscape. COVID was the flood that breached where the levee was, by neglect and design, weakest. It harmed Black and Brown families' health, their wealth, their safety, their mental health.

And the racist history of education helps explain what happened with public schools here during the pandemic: how it is that the United States would become the only wealthy country that in no way prioritized its schools for reopening, losing more cumulative learning days than any other.

But the story of racism is incomplete without the story of resistance. And that's particularly true with education.

For every marginalized group in society—women, enslaved African people and their descendants, Native Americans, Irish Catholic and Chicano immigrants, people with disabilities, gay and trans people—public education has loomed as a civic battleground, as a crucial manifestation of, and as a prerequisite for, basic civil rights and equal participation of all kinds.

And while they fought for an equal place in the public schools, marginalized people have also worked to provide their kids with what they needed on their own, because childhood is short and children can't wait for systems to change. Both of these drives—to be heard within the system and to make a way on one's own—surfaced strongly during the COVID year.

DEMOCRACY AND THE AFRICAN FREE SCHOOL

Black people have always been vocal in US education, even during the time of slavery. In the late 1820s, according to historian John Rury, enrollment in the New York African Free School, founded by the Manumission Society, began to drop even as New York City's Black population was rising. In 1832 the head of school's resignation was suddenly announced. He was a white man named Charles Andrews. The school's trustees reported that the Black community objected to Andrews's support for colonization—that is, sending Black people back to Africa. There was a competing story that Andrews had caned a student for the offense of referring to a Black visitor as a "gentleman."

Whatever the case against Andrews, the Manumission Society acknowledged, "it would be more satisfactory to those who send their children to our schools if a person of their own colour could be obtained competent to conduct a school in a suitable manner." James Adams, a Black teacher, replaced Andrews, and several graduates of the school were hired as teachers. Enrollment rose to new heights.

The community had successfully made its voice heard. Access to school was not sufficient if their children were to be taught by racists. Rury calls this an "unprecedented event," noting, "urban charity schooling was not meant to be democratic."

Unprecedented, rare, and temporary: within the year, the Manumission Society handed the reins of the school over to the Public School Society, making it part of the city's rapidly expanding, taxpayer-supported, and legally segregated education system.

Black teachers and leaders are still underrepresented in public schools centuries later. Today across the country, public school teachers are 80 percent white, while just under half the students are white.

OVERLAYING MAPS OF SLAVERY AND SEGREGATION

I talked to a woman who has been fighting for half a century to secure access to sufficient education, other basic needs, and human rights for

Black children and for all children. She drew me the line from the time of slavery, through her lived experience in the 1960s civil rights movement, to today.

Oleta Fitzgerald, who grew up in Mississippi, directs the southern regional office of the Children's Defense Fund there. CDF advocates for programs for all children living in poverty, like the State Children's Health Insurance Program and Head Start. Fitzgerald's career with the organization goes back to its founding in 1973; she also worked in the Clinton administration.

Marian Wright Edelman was the first Black woman admitted to the Mississippi Bar. She founded the Children's Defense Fund after working with Dr. Martin Luther King on his Poor People's Campaign. "Marian Wright Edelman came out of the civil rights movement. The aggressiveness of the mission and focus, it does inform our work," Fitzgerald tells me. "It's long been understood in the Black community, you know, going back to *Brown v. Board*, and before, going back to slavery, the only way we were going to survive and function was through education... so education as a civil right is something that is infused in the work that we do."

During the pandemic, the southern communities Fitzgerald serves were dealing with job losses and hunger, like other families around the country. Even before that, Mississippi, the poorest state in the union, consistently ranked in the bottom five for spending per public school pupil. Schools didn't have much in the way of technology programs, maybe some computers in the library. The lack of rural broadband service made online schooling especially hard to manage. High school students who had access to cars, Fitzgerald says, would park outside of Walmart or McDonald's to pick up a Wi-Fi signal to do their schoolwork. Often they did this after their own working hours.

Another factor that made online learning especially hard in Mississippi, Fitzgerald says, was the large number of children living with their grandparents. She put me in touch with Shirley Leake, in Jackson, who at the age of eighty-five, was raising the twelve-year-old child of a relative—the last, Leake tells me, of half a dozen she had

...sed. "He's real smart. And sometimes I will ask him about technology stuff that I don't know about. But he'll lie to me about certain things."

Fitzgerald grew up in Mississippi, in Madison County. "If you look at a map across the Deep South, of areas with the highest rates of enslaved people, and they overlay that map with areas of persistent poverty, those maps are almost identical." And it's not such a long way from Jim Crow to now, especially not for those who have lived it. "People who are now above sixty years old," like her, Fitzgerald continues, "would have gone to school in that [pre-*Brown*] system. Their children would be, say, forty. So that's one generation away from not having a public school system, but you still had really bad schools. And then the next generation is the generation that would be in school now."

THE PROBLEM WE ALL LIVE WITH AND THE LITTLE ROCK NINE

The fight to integrate public schools in the 1950s and 1960s has been reduced to a Norman Rockwell painting. Or a cartoon. In 2020, presumably in a response to the country's racial reckoning, Nickelodeon, the children's channel, put out a truly strange animated music video. It starred Ruby Bridges, the poster child of Rockwell's 1963 work *The Problem We All Live With*. She integrated a New Orleans elementary school by herself at the age of six in 1960. In the cartoon, she appears as a purple-haired, singing mermaid, a reference to the Nickelodeon show *Bubble Guppies*. She's accompanied by Peppa Pig on drums. "Ruby was a hero / For you, and me, and everybody!" sings Chris Jackson, who starred as George Washington in the Broadway production of *Hamilton*. Thurgood Marshall, the attorney who argued and won *Brown v. Board of Education* in 1954, has a merman tail too.

Yet integration was no fantasy tale. It was a war, with children on the front lines.

Melba Pattillo Beals is one of the Little Rock Nine who integrated Central High School in Arkansas in 1957. Beals's 2018 memoir *I*

Will Not Fear recounts her having acid sprayed in her eyes and being menaced with lighted sticks of dynamite, a double-barreled shotgun, and a rope. Arkansas governor Orval Faubus called out the National Guard to stop Beals and her classmates. President Dwight Eisenhower responded by sending the 101st Airborne infantry; he also federalized the National Guard to protect the students.

But being inside the school building did not mean safety. At school, students would smear peanut butter full of broken glass shards on her back or under her seat for her to step in. When she went to the restroom, girls lit twists of paper on fire and threw them into her stall, while another girl held the door closed.

Like many a teenage recruit to a cause, Beals started as a true believer. "I naively believed that if we could end segregation in the schools, all barriers of inequality would fall," she told the radio show *Fresh Air*.

The violence and threats tempered her faith into something steelier: the will for survival. "I really had to make a transition in my head. Do you want to live? And what are you willing to do to live? And you're going to have to defend your life every day. Those days of childhood, of sweetness, of being protected by the will of God... there's been a transition here, my darling."

THE LOST YEAR

Beals gave up a lot in that transition. She never graduated from Central High School. There were wanted posters around town with her picture, offering $5,000 for her capture alive and $10,000 for her death. She had to leave her family. The NAACP resettled her with a white couple who were Quaker activists and academics across the country in California. There she finished high school, went on to college and graduate school, and became a journalist and author.

The fall after she first entered school, in August 1958, the Arkansas state legislature passed four laws designed to block desegregation by closing Little Rock's four public high schools, Black and white, entirely. It became known as the Lost Year.

The Lost Year was an example of what Heather McGhee calls in her 2020 book, *The Sum of Us*, "draining the public pool." Her book describes how white Americans time and again will allow the destruction of a public good rather than share that public good with nonwhites. It wasn't the only time this happened: Prince Edward County, in Virginia, also officially closed its public schools for a much longer time, from 1959 to 1964, after being sued in one of the cases decided in *Brown v. Board of Education*. In that case the county used state funds to operate schools for white children.

The Lost Year in Little Rock wasn't lost for everyone. A reported 93 percent of white students in Little Rock managed to attend a private, parochial, or out-of-state public school. Of about 750 Black students displaced, however, half found no schooling at all.

White teachers attempted to hold classes on television. A Women's Emergency Committee to Open Our Schools formed, made up of white upper-class women. People suddenly got very interested in voter registration and school board elections. In May 1959, forty-four teachers were "purged" as suspected integrationists. Schools reopened in the fall only after a federal court ruling. Integration crept along at a token pace for another decade, until the institution of federal busing programs in 1971, which coincided with the beginning of white flight. Today Little Rock Public Schools are 61 percent Black, 19 percent white, and 16 percent Latinx. Suburban Bryant, the highest-regarded school district in the area, is the mirror image: 62 percent white.

THE LOST YEAR AND THE STOLEN YEAR

What can Little Rock's Lost Year tell us about what I am calling the Stolen Year? It's a very different matter, on its face, to close school buildings because of a public health crisis than because of a racist vendetta. But when you think about the forces that kept the majority of the nation's students out of school buildings for the entirety of 2020, particularly in cities, there are connections. Like the social determinants of health that made some communities much harder hit by the pandemic and much more wary to return. Like the lack of trust by families of color that the schools would do what they said they would to keep students safe. Like the continuing disparities in funding that meant buildings serving primarily children of color were older, in worse repair, more crowded, and more poorly ventilated than those serving primarily white students.

There are connections to be found in the unequal impact of closing schools and the unequal responses. Who had computers and Wi-Fi and adults able to help out? Who had money for private school? Who formed emergency committees to open the schools; who organized and lobbied and sued and overturned school board elections, in the absolute conviction that they were entitled to public education on their terms?

Who dropped out, got jobs, got married, cared for younger siblings, and generally had their life courses altered?

The danger that children would be harmed by prolonged school closures in 2020 was clear from the beginning. So was the likelihood that these harms would track existing inequities. As someone who reports on all the valiant efforts of public school educators to right those inequities, I was one of many observers dismayed at what looked like a lack of urgency about reopening in so many places. It seemed like depraved indifference to children's welfare. The Lost Year reveals this isn't the first time that kind of indifference was on display.

But this story also helped me understand something personal that exists in tension with what I just wrote. I am a white woman who attended de facto segregated public schools in 1980s and 1990s Louisiana. I sent my daughters to only slightly less segregated public schools in 2010s Brooklyn. I had a set of inherited assumptions about the inherent benevolence of public education. These assumptions aren't shared by everyone. Just as the resources I take advantage of for my own family aren't shared equally by everyone.

I realized the Norman Rockwell story of schools and the civil rights movement is one white America loves to tell. It's inherently flattering to us because it's about Black people fighting to get into our schools. The cartoon segregationists yelling in the faces of Ruby Bridges and Melba Pattillo Beals feel comfortably foreign to many white people, even though most white people are still sending our children to mostly white schools.

The Norman Rockwell story also doesn't demand that public schools change how or what they teach or who is teaching, only that they change who is sitting in which classroom.

FREEDOM SCHOOLS

But there's another story of the civil rights movement and education, one that also found its echoes in the pandemic. It's the story of freedom schools.

"Freedom schools actually started back in the late '50s, '60s," Oleta Fitzgerald explained to me. "And initially they were designed to teach people about voting and what to say when they went to register to vote. How to answer the questions."

From the 1890s until the Voting Rights Act passed in 1965, some southern states used literacy tests to block Black people's access to the polls. (Before and after the 2020 election, a wave of new "voter fraud" laws passed with similar aims.)

Literacy tests leveraged the historic denial of education rights to block the right to civic participation. Septima Clark, known as the "mother of the movement," was a teacher fired in South Carolina for her membership in the NAACP. She was among those who started citizenship schools to prepare adults for those tests, though many were contrived to be impossible to pass. Clark brought local activists from around the South to the Highlander Folk School in Tennessee, a center established for labor organizing, with communist roots.

Lessons were developed in collaboration with students. The topics spoke to the direct needs of adults who both farmed the land for a living and wanted to vote. "We used the election laws of that particular state to teach the reading. We used the amount of fertilizer and the amount of seeds to teach the arithmetic. . . . We did some political work by having them find out about the kind of government that they had in their particular community. And these were the things that we taught them [to teach] when they went back home," Clark told oral historian Eugene Walker in 1976. "They had to also promise that they would go back to the community and open up a school, and they were supposed to teach two nights a week, two hours each night. We had all of the books mimeographed that we wanted them to use in teaching." Clark was known for the slogan "literacy means liberation."

Building on the citizenship school model, activists began to start "freedom schools" to teach children as well as adults. The idea: Give people the knowledge and skills to make change. Teach them history, especially their own history, so they know how change is made. And give them the respect and attention—the care and the love—to make them believe that they can make change.

Freedom schools appeared in Prince Edward County, Virginia, during its own segregationist school closures from 1959 to 1964. They happened during public school boycotts in New York City, Chicago, and Boston in the early 1960s. And during the Freedom Summer in Mississippi in 1964, when the Student Nonviolent Coordinating Committee brought several hundred white college students down to the state to volunteer to register voters. An aspiring writer named Charles Cobb and a former New York City teacher named Robert Moses were among those who got the idea to open a school using the student volunteers as teachers (particularly the women—this was gendered work). Septima Clark, Ella Baker, and Bayard Rustin came together with other activists and academics in New York City to write a curriculum that covered civics, citizenship, the history of nonviolence, and Black history. The schools also offered electives, like guitar, dance, French, poetry, and auto mechanics.

According to historian Daniel Perlstein, eventually forty-one schools opened around Mississippi, with nearly two thousand students ranging in age from four years old to twenty-five. Students and teachers sometimes spent their mornings learning and their after-noons together registering voters and picketing. The philosophy was as egalitarian and progressive as possible. "It was like a community-driven education system," remembers Fitzgerald. "And some people say it did better [than school] in terms of molding and then working with the whole child. It wasn't just about grades and learning. It was about developing young people."

LIBERATION AND LITERACY

The COVID "lost year" of school spawned its own efforts toward alternative education. Some of them exceeded their emergency purpose and became liberatory. This happened in homes, in neighborhood pods or micro-schools, and in traditional classrooms gone virtual. In Seattle, during the spring, Jesse Hagopian brought teaching artists to talk to his students over Zoom about oppression and the legacy of trauma through hip-hop and Native American folklore. He taught them about Septima Clark and Ella Baker too. "I've been trying to give historical context so that they can learn from the struggles of the past and then apply those lessons today."

The Children's Defense Fund has its own summer enrichment program, in partnership with community organizations, called Freedom Schools. It was severely scaled back during the pandemic but still served twenty-five hundred children nationwide in the summer of 2020. None, however, were in Mississippi. When I spoke to Fitzgerald, she was excited about returning in the summer of 2021. "We know that we've got to do something like MASH units to try to get these kids back, to regain what they need—not only the learning loss but also the mental anguish."

Meanwhile out in Oakland, California, where the Black Panthers had started their own community-based school project as well as their school breakfast program, a social entrepreneur named Laki-sha Young remade her entire organization in response to COVID, launching another Freedom School–inspired program.

Young is a single mother of three and a first-generation college graduate who grew up in the Bay Area. She founded the Oakland Reach originally to organize low-income Black and Brown parents to push policymakers for school reforms. It was an organization directed at developing a voice in education, in other words.

She often points out that in Oakland, only 30 percent of Black and Hispanic students were reading at grade level, and that was before the pandemic. "We are trying to disrupt an educational system that has put our kids in a pipeline...that has really exacerbated intergenerational poverty," she told me. "When you think about community organizing, you have to choose something that's very important to the people that you're organizing, and so that's opportunity and their kids' futures, in this case."

Then the pandemic hit. Oakland Unified School District switched to virtual learning. Twitter founder Jack Dorsey donated $10 million to the district's students to buy devices, yet at the end of the school year, a reported five thousand students were still left without computers. Students were catching Wi-Fi signals in school parking lots and getting limited live instruction.

"We were surveying and listening to our families, and what we were hearing was loss of connection with their teachers," said Young. "They didn't have the infrastructure to support any kind of robust virtual learning—bad internet, old computers, not enough computers."

In this context, signing petitions and holding rallies didn't make sense to Young anymore. Her organization pivoted from voice to direct aid. It raised a $400,000 relief fund to help about a thousand of its families with small direct grants for basic needs: rent, groceries, utilities.

On the national level, she saw handwringing, but ultimately complacency, about the pandemic's disproportionate impact on Black and Brown kids. "It was kind of like sitting at the kitchen table and being like, OK, no one's coming to save us. Right? And we must design and create the solutions. We're on the ground. We know what's happening. We need to create a model that really supports our families."

In June 2020, as her teenage daughter was taking part in BLM protests in Oakland, Young launched a summer learning program. She partnered with a local internet café and tech repair shop to put working devices in the hands of children who didn't have them. And she recruited fourteen local teachers to run online summer school classes for K–8 students, with live video teaching in basic subjects, plus enrichment like art and music. She called it the Literacy Liberation Center.

It was small. It was voluntary. But it worked well for the two hundred students who participated. They progressed an average of two reading levels, according to the district's assessment. The instruction was part of a free nationwide effort called the National Summer School Initiative, started and funded mostly by people from the charter school and education reform movement. The larger initiative enrolled about fifteen thousand students during the summer across the country, offering several hours a day of live instruction and enrichment.

The Reach also hired some mothers from the community directly to serve as "family liaisons," helping others navigate not only online learning but housing, employment, and aid options.

Toni Rochelle, one of these liaisons, had moved to the area with two small children after going through a difficult divorce. She was placed on administrative leave from her job just before COVID. "I hadn't had a paycheck from my job in three months," she told me. "I think we all were kind of like in a panic and a shock trying to get adjusted to everything. "

The Reach gave her family computers, helped out with rent, and signed her son and daughter up for the summer program. "I can tell the difference of the special care that they're getting from the hub versus school," she said. "I love all the teachers there. They were so patient. Like grandmothers—loving, nurturing people. It wasn't a big classroom. So they were able to give individual care."

Then they hired Toni to help other families. "I was a parent that was freaking out and I was trying to figure out stuff. And then all of a sudden I became a parent and an advocate to help other parents so they wouldn't freak out like I was."

In the crisis, the Reach, like community-based organizations all over the country, changed its tactics. It morphed from a pressure group, petitioning the powers that be for change, into a little echo of the nineteenth-century settlement houses or a Black Panther "survival pending revolution" project: employment and training for mothers, learning for children, basic needs for all.

Reach Learning Hubs expanded in the fall, partnering more extensively with the school district. "What it's also becoming is a way for parents to start to see what they deserve and should receive around their kids' education," Young mused. "Because business as usual has been interrupted, and now people can start to see the holes in the underwear. And so instead of trying to turn them back to a system that's been failing them, let's design the thing that we would want to see for ourselves."

Lakisha Young isn't Septima Clark. She's no Communist, for one thing. Reach has been criticized since its founding as an Astroturf, or fake grassroots, organization. It gets its money from organizations like the Center on Reinventing Public Education, whose backers include Mark Zuckerberg, Bill Gates, and the Waltons, of Walmart fame. These funders are known for pressing for a slate of school reforms that traditional public school advocates, like teacher unions, criticize as a path to privatization. They include more charter schools, stricter accountability rules, and a bigger role for technology, data, and standardized testing.

As an organizer and activist herself, Young could acknowledge that the rap against her was "a very powerful message": "These billionaire funders are trying to come in here, these privatizers trying to take over." She rejects the premise of applying a "purity test" to her funding. "It's really racist to suggest that groups give us money and tell us what to do," she said. "We are powerful leaders and parents— we use the money to do what parents want and need. No funder shifts our purpose."

Accountability, Young points out, goes both ways. "We gotta take a long and hard look at union agreements which uphold a status quo where our kids can't fucking read!"

Despite these fighting words, she calls her relationship with the district "pretty good." They partnered to expand the learning hub in the 2020–2021 school year. She said her whole effort has been concentrated around the question "How do we push this model into the system?" The push was pretty strong: Reach went on to join a lawsuit against Oakland Unified for denial of an adequate online education, which I'll get to in Chapter 11.

When public school buildings went quiet in 2020, it left a space to think about what had been going on there, what might have been, and what could be. Some people wanted to get back to normal as fast as possible. Others believed, for good reason, that normal had never been good enough. And that divide would continue to dog the school years to come.

THE SCARECROWS

Back on the East Coast, on June 2, Patricia was facing down a phalanx of cops and armed anti–Black Lives Matter counterprotesters as she tried to get her son to the hospital. "I was sitting there arguing [with the police]. They're saying a motorcade is coming through and I'm telling them, no, I need to go that way. I need it. My son needs to get COVID tested, today, so I can have him on the [operating] table by the 4th. They were trying to tow my car. I said I'm not moving."

PJ, her five-year-old, wanted to know what was going on. "I was explaining to him that these people were protesting. I was trying to explain to him and drive the car and figure out what was going on." PJ and his parents had come up with a word that helped him be less afraid of empty-headed white people acting angry, whether he saw them on the streets or on TV: "He kept saying, 'Oh, Mommy, they're just scarecrows,'...because the scarecrow doesn't have a brain." But as the confrontation wore on, he started crying from fear in the backseat.

Patricia wasn't having it. "I was like, NO. Sometimes in life you have to stand on what you believe in. Keep your mask on. Sit there, don't move. You're about to watch Mommy get her way."

And she did. "Finally, they let me through and they gave me an escort to the hospital."

6 COURTS

In Germany, Denmark, Norway, Sweden, and many other countries, SCHOOLS ARE OPEN WITH NO PROBLEMS. The Dems think it would be bad for them politically if U.S. schools open before the November election, but it is important for the children & families. May cut off funding if not open!

—Trump, Twitter, July 8, 2020

It's like, you'll go, "Person, woman, man, camera, TV." So, they'd say, "Could you repeat that?" So, I said, "Yeah—person, woman, man, camera, TV."

—Trump, describing taking a cognitive test on Fox News, July 22, 2020

June 30, 2020, with 4 percent of the global population, the US has 25 percent of the global coronavirus cases and the second-highest death rate per capita

July 7, 2020, US death toll passes 130,000

It was the summer of 2020. Online classes had, mercifully, ended for the year. In San Francisco, Jonah and his mom no longer had to go through the daily dance of slammed laptops and yelling.

Maya finally found out what was wrong with *her* mom, Jonah's grandma, who had been feeling ill. It was lung cancer. Severe, stage four.

While Maya was trying to deal with this blow and coordinate her mother's care, Jonah's friend Khamla reached out by text.

They hadn't seen Khamla since the spring, when Robert, Maya's partner, had dropped a school computer off at Khamla's house for remote learning. Khamla's father, who is older and only speaks Lao, was belligerent—apparently suspicious that it was some kind of scam.

Khamla's text to Maya said, "How are you guys doing?"

Maya replied, "Good. What's going on? How's your family?"

"Not so great," Khamla replied.

He texted a blurry picture that was hard to make out at first. It was a piece of broken furniture.

Maya contacted a local organization that works with Southeast Asian immigrants to try to get help for Khamla. The caseworker there encouraged her to call Child Protective Services, or CPS. "I've never called CPS. I don't know what that means. And I'm not much of a crier, and I literally start sobbing on the phone with her. And she was lovely and held the space for me. I just think that was, like, a lot about my mom, because I'm crying to her and I say, I can't take Khamla away from his mom."

WHAT CAN SEPARATE A FAMILY

This chapter is about the particular COVID experiences of children like Khamla, who are taken away—separated from their families of origin, temporarily or permanently.

The phrase "family separation" might call to mind the thousands of children deliberately separated from their families at the US border with Mexico during the Trump administration.

But that is only one sliver in a heap of broken shards.

In the United States in the years leading up to the pandemic, there were between 425,000 and 435,000 children in the child welfare system, living with foster families and in group homes.

About forty-three thousand teenagers are locked up in the juvenile justice system (including some forty-five hundred in adult jails and prisons).

And, another seven hundred thousand teenagers also spend some time each year on their own without stable housing. They are sometimes known as "runaways," sometimes "throwaways." They often intersect with the legal system as they try to survive.

THE ARCHIPELAGO

These systems of child separation have common historical origins. These origins are dark. They are rooted in slavery, colonialism, anti-immigrant sentiment, and the genocide and dispossession of Native Americans.

As the academic and advocate Laura Briggs argues in *Taking Children: A History of American Terror*, the US government has been routinely separating children who are not white, who are recent immigrants, and who are poor from their kin for four hundred years. And as her subtitle argues, the core reasons are often political.

These systems are connected. One study found that youth aging out of foster care had up to a 46 percent chance of experiencing homelessness in their young adulthood. A 2019 survey by the *Kansas City Star* found that one-quarter of all prisoners nationwide had been in foster care. Immigrant families, like Khamla's, are more likely to have encounters with the child welfare system and difficulties navigating it.

They are connected to other structures of injustice too. According to a 2017 study that followed half a million children born in California, one in four children were the subject of a child welfare services investigation during their childhood. For Black and Native American families, the figure was startlingly higher, more than one in two.

You see this same disparity in the juvenile justice system: Black youth are five times as likely to be incarcerated as white youth, and Native youth are three times as likely.

These complex and interlocking systems of family and youth separation and control remind me of *The Gulag Archipelago*. The book is a blend of memoir and reporting by the Nobel Prize–winning Russian dissident Aleksandr Solzhenitsyn. It is set in the network of prisons and forced labor camps that grew up under communism.

Although it uses terms like "welfare," "social services," and "rehabilitation," the United States operates what many people familiar with the system would characterize as a gulag archipelago for children.

I know that sounds shocking, so let me explain.

This archipelago is not solely made up of literal prisons, jails, and detention centers—only partly.

It includes airless visiting rooms with tiled floors, long hallways, steel file cabinets full of dusty paperwork. And sometimes cheerful group homes and loving, welcoming individual family foster homes.

It's not dedicated to torture, but physical and emotional abuse are too likely to occur. It's not intentionally designed for political repression, but the children who are part of this system are too often elided in our policymaking and forgotten. And they are very likely to belong to populations that are already marginalized.

Above all, it's a vast bureaucracy that depends for its power on citizen surveillance.

For totalitarian regimes to be effective, neighbors, colleagues, and loved ones must be willing to inform on each other.

When it comes to the children's archipelago, state "mandatory reporter" laws draft tens of millions of people into the role of potential informant. Doctors, teachers, and counselors must report all suspected maltreatment of children. In eighteen states the mandatory reporting obligation extends to all adults.

By making that call, you can ensure a family gets investigated but not that they get helped.

During the pandemic, children in what I'm calling the archipelago were affected in similar and revealing ways.

Many were denied in-person visits with their families, sometimes for a full year.

Some were put on lockdown for COVID quarantine, which at times amounted to solitary confinement.

Some had limited access to education. They missed other services, too, like recreation, vocational training, and therapy.

Finally and surprisingly, the working of these systems was slowed and altered by lockdown, sometimes in ways that made reformers, including those who call themselves abolitionists, optimistic about the future.

QUARANTINE IN A CHURCH BASEMENT

Mala left her father's house, which she describes as a "toxic environment," for an LGBTQ youth shelter on the Upper West Side of Manhattan in March 2020. "It's coming to a point where I have to realize neither of my parents are really willing to help me," she said. "They're not really treating me like family, and it was time for me to accept that and actually move on."

The shelter was in a church basement. In normal times there are fourteen residents, who are asked to leave by 6:00 a.m. and come back at 8:00 p.m. Because of the pandemic, the number of beds was cut in half. Mala was asked to sign a paper saying she would go nowhere except for an hour walk in Riverside Park once a day. It sunk in that she was going on lockdown with half a dozen strangers.

Still, she believed she had made the right choice. "Imagine if I would have stayed with my dad.... I couldn't even fathom how my father would even help support me, or even cared. Even though I'm surrounded by more people at the shelter, instead of being in an apartment with my parent and me just being in my own room and him having his own room, it still felt like I was in a better situation being in a shelter."

Across the country, a major reason youth like Mala can't live at home any longer is that their families are homophobic or transphobic. Young people with LGBTQ identities are by some estimates more than twice as likely to be on the streets, in shelters, or couch surfing.

The pandemic was a crisis for these young people several times over. They lost the support of school and community groups. Social distancing requirements and staff limitations meant fewer beds.

Many cities, including New York, took steps to house more homeless people during COVID in hotels and similar places. But for teenagers there was more red tape. They had to go through a lengthy referral process. "So think of a kid who's homeless that is scared and sick in the middle of a pandemic, sitting in an office somewhere, sometimes for up to two days, isolated by themselves until they get picked up to be brought to a hotel," Jamie Powlovich, director of the Empire State Coalition of Youth and Family Services, told me.

Many of Mala's fellow residents, whom the shelter called clients, had trouble with the strict rules at the shelter. "People weren't really understanding the concept [of lockdown]. They felt that we were having to be subjected to martial law. And some clients were making comments that, oh, I have work to do, which really meant, I have to go to Times Square and ask people for money, or be on the train all day."

There were fights and tantrums. Cops were called. Some of her roommates used racist language against her. Mala also thought the way the staff treated them was demeaning. She withdrew and didn't talk much. "Some of these conversations...can escalate really quickly. My peers tended to, like, black out and rant about things and it can get out of hand. I was pretty traumatized and scared," she said.

Things got worse after a few weeks, in April, when she came down with what she describes as a bad flu. She never got a COVID test. Since the shelter was all one room, the staff tried to quarantine her by putting her bed on the church basement's small stage. She was lying on her cot, cut off by a thick velvet curtain, coughing, dust motes swirling in the air. Her roommates regularly barged across the stage to get out the back door to the small indoor courtyard, which was the only place they could be outside save for one hour a day.

Mala was laid off from her job at a pharmacy at the start of lockdown; with it went some of her hope for a better future. "I remember hearing the pots and pans and the whistles being blown as the essential workers came home, it was really like, wow, this is really happening. And it just made me even more depressed, especially when I had to quarantine myself, and also being sick and me just being so confused, like, I don't know how I'm going to recover from this pandemic or where I'm going to be after shelter because I don't really have any resources, and I'm homeless, and it just doesn't make sense."

LOCKDOWN IN LOCKUP

When the pandemic lockdowns were called, David was finishing up a four-year sentence at the Swanson Center for Youth in Monroe, Louisiana, that began when he was seventeen.

David, who, unlike most juveniles incarcerated in Louisiana, is white, was convicted of aggravated rape. Two years on, his sentence was up for modification. His parents paid for a private lawyer, and his victim testified in favor of his release. The judge, however, upheld the full sentence.

The number of youth incarcerated around the country has been dropping dramatically because of reforms: 60 percent from 2000 to 2017. But Louisiana historically has some of the highest rates of incarceration in the world, and it ranks fifteenth in the nation for its incarceration of juveniles.

At Swanson, David didn't get in trouble. He finished high school and started taking welding classes. "I fell in love with it. I think it's really cool, how it happens. I don't know how to describe it."

His parents have been married forty-two years. David's their youngest and they dote on him. They used to drive eight hours round-trip and stay the night to see him every single weekend. Eventually he was granted weekend furloughs home, then four- and five-day furloughs. They always cooked his favorite foods for him—crawfish boils, steak and potatoes.

When COVID hit, David was home on one of these furloughs, looking forward to fishing for bass and going "mudding" on all-terrain vehicles with his buddies.

Then the call came: David had to return immediately. David's mother could feel him withdraw over the course of the four-hour drive, steeling himself for what was to come. "On the last two hours back to Monroe, he got very, very quiet. He just had to get his mind set into where he was going back."

For her part, she was afraid. "And my husband and I—I could just tear up even just thinking about it....We did not let him know our feelings because I didn't want him upset. But of course, he knew...and, I mean, we all three of us cried when we left."

"When I walked in the gate, they just took my temperature and sent me back to the dorm," David said. Soon his dorm, with seven boys, was put on lockdown. "We were just stuck in a dorm for three weeks, twenty-four hours a day, and we couldn't go nowhere." The bunks were so close together you could graze someone with your knuckles when you turned over in your sleep. The days dragged; they watched TV, slept, played board games. David tried to stay out of arguments, especially over politics.

Starting in March 2020, the facility banned in-person visits for a full year. This happened at secure facilities for youth all over the country.

If my child were locked up, I can imagine that like David's parents, I would want to visit them as much as I could. Research going back to the 1980s shows that incarcerated young people who get to see their families regularly show less depression, better behavior, and are less likely to get arrested again after they are released. However, these findings are confounded, because children from families that are not able to support them consistently with in-person visits might have a harder time for lots of reasons.

Considering that juvenile justice is nominally committed to rehabilitation, you might think that preserving contact with family as much as possible would be a priority. But no. It's common for teenagers to be incarcerated hours away from home, and many never get visits at all. This lack of consideration for family ties has historical roots. Beginning in the nineteenth century, the juvenile justice system, a separate category of urban almshouses and rural reform schools, was founded on the principle of *parens patriae*—the state is stepping in for parents who, it is implied, have failed at their jobs.

Zoom visits were introduced at Swanson in April but weren't always available. David's mother would give him money sometimes to put on his friends' phone accounts, especially some whose family members had gotten COVID.

"You're used to them coming and everything," he told me about the loss of visits. "It just took a toll on you, you're down all the time. Your stress levels are rising because you don't get to see your family. With COVID going on, you want to be able to see them...in case something happens."

"We talked every single day, two or three times a day on the phone, and you could just hear more anger," said his mother. "This one particular time—he's never spoken to me in the voice that he spoke to me. He called me back after an hour or two later and just apologized to me and said, 'Mom, I'm so sorry.'"

Some of his fellow youths escaped during these early days. David said they were desperate to know if their families were OK. "They didn't know what the heck to think," he told me for NPR. "They're not hearing nothing but just the news. And I mean, they talk to their family every now and then, but they want to be with their family when stuff like this happens. They want to be *with* them." In Bridge City, another juvenile facility in Louisiana, there was a riot in April 2020 that sent a staff member to the hospital.

At some institutions, quarantines meant solitary confinement. In recent years, states have begun to limit or prohibit the solitary confinement of teenagers because it's considered a form of child abuse. In 2016, President Obama banned the practice in federal prisons because of the "potential for devastating, lasting psychological consequences."

But during COVID, health concerns took precedence. For example, in December 2020, a COVID outbreak at the juvenile jail in New Orleans meant some teenagers who had not yet been tried or sentenced were confined to their cells for two weeks, some of them all alone.

Incarcerated teenagers are required by law to get schooling, although they're not legally entitled to see their mothers. Between quarantines and a lack of computers and internet access, education faltered in many places during the pandemic. Forty students in the Washington, DC, jail sued the city for providing nothing but paper packets for weeks on end.

David didn't trust Swanson to keep him safe from COVID. Staff members, he heard, were getting it. They gave the youth one disposable mask per day, but he didn't see the point because everyone took them off to shower. "We basically were letting them know, y'all need to give us more masks. And they never did. So we kind of never wore them." Overall, just shy of four thousand COVID infections were reported among incarcerated juveniles and staff members in forty-one states from March 2020 to March 2021.

Eventually, David was let out about a month early, in September 2020. In some ways the outside world felt less secure than inside. "In there, you kind of know where each other've been and everything. But when you come out here, you've got to kind of watch your surroundings and watch who you're around." He started working in his dad's landscaping business and aimed to resume his welding.

Unrest continued at Swanson through the spring of 2021. In May six inmates attacked two guards and escaped. In June an escapee was accused of carjacking. The state said it was giving guards panic buttons. And it was breaking ground on a new $24 million facility within the fence line of the century-old complex. Advocates argued that the state should be closing youth prisons, not building new ones.

David told me that he felt like the juvenile justice system wasn't living up to its promise during the pandemic. "My mom sent me a book to read about the juvenile justice system. It says that we are meant to be rehabilitated and after we have been rehabilitated, we need to be released." Being rehabilitated, he says, means, "you complete your program, and you go six months or a year without getting in trouble, and you're becoming more like a law-abiding citizen. You help out, you take leadership roles. You can see the growth. They start growing into basically a young man, not a child like they were." Cut off from family, it was that much harder to do that, David said. "That's what helps a lot of people up—the support of their family."

ALONE IN A ROOM

COVID isolated and separated people all over the world. For children in the archipelago, it intensified their existing isolation and separation. Because of COVID transmission fears, many foster kids, just like incarcerated kids, were denied in-person visits with their families of origin.

Joyce McMillan, who advocates for families in the foster care system in New York City, told me that the biggest grief visited on them by the pandemic was Zoom-only visitation, which continued for more than a year. "It's torturous for a child to see their parents on-screen, already missing them, unable to see them, hug them, kiss them. Babies scratching the cold, hard screen, trying to reach their parents." The mandated length of a typical weekly visit is two hours, but through a screen, parents couldn't hope to keep small children's attention for more than a fraction of that, so their effective contact time was cut even further.

An attorney in California, speaking to me on background, was saddened by the case of a young mother who had her newborn removed from her care in the hospital because she failed a drug test. She found a bed in a residential treatment facility that allowed children. But the foster parent refused to allow the baby to stay with her there even for short visits, because of the risk of COVID. "Research shows that it's good for mothers' recovery if the babies are with them.... [I]t also helps the baby and it helps development," the attorney said.

Parents who fall under the judgment of family court have to earn their children back by completing a series of onerous quests. These may include commitments like drug rehab, parenting classes, counseling, or a search for housing or a job.

They may progress from supervised visits, to unsupervised visits, to longer and overnight visits, on the path toward regaining custody of their children. When in-person visits weren't happening, they often couldn't make progress, stranded on the other side of the chasm from reunification.

The ban on visitation during COVID also affected the estimated 2.7 million children who have at least one parent incarcerated, as well as youths in residential facilities. The latter includes those with disabilities or psychiatric conditions, some of whom could not be made to understand why their families had apparently abandoned them.

BORDER KIDS

The effects of the pandemic on migrant children would be a whole other book. Thousands were living in camps on the border in Mexico when the border was effectively sealed. Aid and legal resources slowed to a trickle. Kidnappings, assault, and other crimes were rampant.

"They become more traumatized, really, than any children I've seen in my over thirty years of working in vulnerable populations of traumatized children," Amy Cohen told me. She is a psychiatrist who advocates for migrant children and founded the organization Every Last One. During the early months of the pandemic she was evaluating children in Matamoros, Mexico, over FaceTime for the few immigration asylum appeals that could be pursued. "All of them developed night terrors. Some of them became mute, did not speak at all."

Cohen told me, and I confirmed with another advocate who had knowledge of the situation, that during the pandemic, children detained in the United States after crossing the border were sometimes quarantined all alone. "These are children as young as three, four, or five years old. Many are placed in rooms by themselves with no diversions and sometimes nothing but crayons and paper," Cohen said. "The psychological damage to these children who are left by themselves in strange facilities, having been separated from their families, for days and weeks at a time, is very disturbing."

EMERGENCY REMOVAL

Maya believes it was a neighbor of Khamla's who did eventually call Child Protective Services. Toward the end of July, a social worker called and asked whether they would consider taking Khamla in— the very next day. The county was doing an emergency removal of Khamla, an only child, from his home.

They felt conflicted. Not because they had full-time jobs, a child in special education, and an ailing parent already on their plate. Maya and Robert are the type of people who seem to live out their ideals and commitments without question. They were conflicted because they felt Khamla really belonged with his own family, another Lao-speaking family, or at least one who was Asian American.

"I was really clear with them that we knew that the best place for Khamla was with his family, but that we wanted to be here for him and provide whatever support he needed, up to and including permanent placement with us," Maya said.

Ultimately, she was convinced they were Khamla's best option. "We had a relationship with him, his mom had been supportive of us, and then Khamla reached out to us. So it felt like we were responding in a way to a request for help from him and his family." Her instincts were aligned with what is considered best practice today by child welfare reformers: kinship placements are best, cultural alignment is desirable, and family friends are better than strangers.

Jonah was elated. "I needed a friend!" he told his mom.

Robert's son from his first marriage, Rust, had just graduated high school and decided to defer college for a year. He was moving into his mother's garage apartment in the East Bay. So there was some space opening up in their little house with a rose garden on the hill.

Jonah and Khamla wanted to share Jonah's bedroom. "Khamla's whole family was in one room before that. It would be very weird for him to be by himself. He would have been scared," said Maya. "And for Jonah, it was like, 'I want to be with my friend.' It was very cute."

There's an inherent skew to this story; I'm writing about a foster placement from the point of view of the host family. Khamla's parents could not be reached for comment. His mother was living in a shelter during this time, working on getting permanent housing so that Khamla could move back in with her. Maya and Robert weren't supposed to contact her directly. Her caseworker confirmed some details of her case but didn't agree to relay a request for an interview. Neither did her lawyer.

Maya and Robert set up a twin bed from IKEA with dresser drawers underneath, and Khamla moved in at the end of July, the same week that Maya's mother underwent surgery.

The doctor called Maya before her mother was even awake from the anesthesia to deliver the bad news; the cancer had spread too many places to be effectively removed. When Maya's mother woke up, she was alone in the hospital because of COVID. She had to absorb the news with no family to hold her hand.

DIMMING OF THE SEARCHLIGHTS

I've been describing the impacts of the pandemic on children within the archipelago. But COVID also narrowed the channels into the system. It reduced scrutiny of families.

Advocates hope that this might be an opening to reimagine the workings of the archipelago altogether.

Courts and other bureaucracies generally slowed down. For some families it meant they couldn't make any progress toward reunifying with their children, or getting a juvenile's appeal heard. For others it was a good thing; it meant postponing a deportation, for example.

During COVID, child welfare was less intrusive. Inspection visits sometimes came over Zoom instead of to the front door. Many families were relieved: "They're not opening my refrigerator. They're not opening my dresser drawers. They're not strip-searching my children and they're not asking me to take their clothes off for the camera, because that would be child pornography," as Joyce McMillan, the family advocate in New York City, told Bloomberg News.

Youth arrests, particularly the tens of thousands that occur at schools every year, fell. Overall the population of incarcerated youth decreased by a third during the pandemic, mostly because fewer young people entered the system in March and April.

In some states, including Pennsylvania, Louisiana, and Maryland, families sued to get their children released from secure facilities during the pandemic. In Maryland they prevailed, but in Louisiana the state Office of Juvenile Justice successfully argued that they were balancing public health and rehabilitation the best they could.

Hailly Korman is an expert on youth justice reform at Bellwether Education Partners, a nonprofit consultancy. She told me for NPR that she saw the drop in youth incarceration during COVID as an opportunity. "If it was OK to close these buildings because kids didn't need to be in them, and we're just as safe as we were before...that tells us something about the utility of these institutions."

CHILD WELFARE DATA VOID

It's not entirely clear that families or communities were "just as safe as before" during the pandemic. There was a spike in homicides and in drug overdoses, both of which affected young people.

Some public health experts also forecast a spike in child abuse and domestic violence. The two are often linked, as in the case of Khamla's family. Families were absolutely seeing more hardship and stress, which are risk factors for neglect and abuse, respectively. Previous natural disasters led to a rise in reported abuse.

Alicia Lieberman holds an endowed chair in infant mental health at the University of California and focuses on young and traumatized children.

While it wasn't the sole cause of any incident, "COVID creates a context that increases the risk of child maltreatment," Lieberman told me. "More fighting, more depression, more anxiety, more likely to lose patience with the children…or neglect if a parent needs to work." And parents lost access to support from family, friends, and church, even stress relievers like exercise.

However, data did not conclusively reveal more child abuse across the country during the pandemic. Domestic violence reports to police rose between 10 and 27 percent in various jurisdictions in the first weeks of lockdown. But official reports to child protection agencies fell between 20 and 70 percent across the country.

Out of millions of emergency room visits nationwide, the total number in which child abuse or neglect was suspected dropped from March to October 2020 compared to the year before. But, among those who were identified as possible victims, the comparatively small number who had injuries severe enough to actually admit them to the hospital remained the same as the year before. In New York City, the commissioner of the Administration for Children's Services (ACS) said that emergency room trends were unchanged and concluded, "we really haven't seen any indicators" of an increase in undetected child abuse. The unsettling truth, however, is that when it comes to child maltreatment during the pandemic, we just don't know what we don't know.

EDUCATIONAL NEGLECT

Even as overall reports to child welfare went down in 2020, some families were reported specifically because of the pandemic. In June, a coalition of child advocates in New York City sent a letter to the city's public advocate, Jumaane Williams, complaining about schools calling child welfare to report families who were having trouble with remote learning for "educational neglect."

Their clients included families in homeless shelters who were having trouble getting Wi-Fi and families with language barriers who didn't understand the school's log-in instructions. One parent had the school's remote learning device shipped to the wrong address and was reported while she waited for a new one. In another case, a school called ACS on a family whose child was logging in to remote learning daily and completing all of his coursework but had a technical problem submitting that work to the teacher. The letter noted that besides these reports being intimidating and triggering or prolonging investigations, they can lead to parents being placed on a statewide registry of child abusers, which makes it difficult to find a job. Arguably the schools were using child welfare to cast blame on the families they had failed to help. This issue continued into the fall of 2021, when New York City schools opened up with no remote option; families who still feared in-person school had child welfare called on them.

A DIFFERENT KIND OF SYSTEM

It's perfectly possible to imagine a drop in child abuse reports that doesn't conceal a hidden epidemic of abuse. That's because an estimated 80 to 90 percent of child abuse and neglect reports are not ultimately substantiated.

Rates of substantiated child maltreatment have been falling at least since the early 1990s.

By far the most common cause of a child welfare report is neglect, which usually ties in some way to poverty: children outside without shoes or no car seat when it's time to bring a baby home from the hospital. And child poverty has been on the rise. In 2018, one in four children entered the system because of neglect alone.

And yet state Child Protective Services agencies typically have more money to spend investigating and monitoring families and removing children than they do on assistance to families. A foster parent gets a monthly child support payment from the state, but that kind of payment historically hasn't been available to parents to support their own children.

A fascinating paper looked at trends in child removal in Florida from March through the end of June 2020, compared with previous years.

Overall, the number of children placed in foster care fell by more than one-fifth. Proportionately fewer Black children were taken away for what the researchers termed more discretionary reasons, such as neglect, inadequate supervision, or parental substance abuse. Meanwhile, proportionately more white children were removed because of serious, substantiated claims of maltreatment, such as physical and sexual abuse.

This is one study in one state. But it paints a picture of a system that could be less racially disproportionate and more focused on the most serious cases.

Can we make families and communities safer, without over-policing? This question goes to the heart of the debate over the child archipelago.

"NO ONE WAS HELPING ME"

When her son was shot, Heather, who you met in Chapter 3, lost custody of her first two children, who were born when she was, in her words, a "hard-headed teenager." She's retained her rights over her remaining eight children, although at times she's lived in her car and in housing that didn't have enough space for all of them or didn't have running water or working major appliances.

During the pandemic she was living in a small duplex with only one bathroom. Sometimes the children stayed with their fathers, other family, or friends. They've also spent stints at Annie Malone, which is a rare type of private nonprofit home in St. Louis that offers respite care. Children whose housing is up in the air or who have psychological or behavioral problems can stay there temporarily without automatically initiating the process of investigating or terminating their parents' rights. Access to this kind of short-term care has been shown to reduce parent stress along with removal of children from their families. Annie Malone's chief development officer, Jarel Loveless, said they are dedicated to helping families before they get "hotlined," or reported to the Department of Social Services. The agency served more than five hundred families during the pandemic.

When seven-year-old Habersham was shot, the incident triggered a child welfare investigation from St. Louis's Department of Social Services, or DSS.

"I had to deal with DSS for six weeks. They felt like I was neglecting my son or something." This was while childcares in her neighborhood had closed. So had schools. Heather was trying to support her family on a ten-dollar-an-hour job at a homeless shelter. "The people I counted on to help me, they didn't. The people that were coming here for six weeks, they kept on telling me to do floor time," that is, get down on the floor and play with her children—generic parenting advice. "And I'm like, I need your help! They never were bringing me the things that I needed."

Heather was proud of her children's loyalty and affection. When the social service investigators asked to talk to the children alone, Heather told them, fine. She wasn't worried what they'd say; she'd use the time to go to Walmart. "They told them, 'My momma loves me. I eat every day. I get everything I need. I don't have all my wants, but I have all my needs.'" DSS ultimately closed the investigation.

But she still felt wounded and judged—by the officials, and by her friends and family. "When COVID first started there wasn't any outlet for the children, no places for them to play," she says. "When [the shooting] happened everyone was on my case, like, 'oh, these kids need help.' But no one was helping me." In fact, she remained without childcare and even worse off than before. Because of the social services investigation, she was now scared to lock the door on her kids, and she started to be late to work. On June 28, 2020, she was fired.

STRAY KITTENS

Throughout this book I've described moments where child policy in the United States turned away from supporting families and toward maligning, punishing, and separating them.

For example, in 1912, when Julia Lathrop became the first head of the Children's Bureau, and the first woman to head any federal agency, she took up "orphanage, juvenile courts, desertion" rather than mothers' income supports—a nascent state-level initiative at that time—or subsidized childcare. Or in the mid-1940s, when the federal government shut down the childcare program that had been set up to aid the World War II effort, New York City's welfare commissioner, Edward E. Rhatigan, threatened working mothers with foster care. Or in 1996, as part of the Contract with America, when Republican House Speaker Newt Gingrich suggested cutting welfare benefits to unwed teen mothers and using that money to put their children in orphanages instead.

People in power continue to decide that it's morally preferable to "rescue" children like so many kittens, punishing their parents by separating them. It's an extension of the delusion perpetuated by Victorian "hidden mother" photography—that it's somehow feasible on a broad scale to have thriving children without thriving families of origin.

CHILD TAKING AS A FORM OF TERRORISM

Think of the central image of the bestselling 1852 abolitionist novel *Uncle Tom's Cabin*: Eliza crossing a frozen river to save her babe in arms from being sold away from her. Taking children was the emblematic cruelty of chattel slavery.

Enslaved people rarely had to contend with claims that their children were being taken for their own good. This wasn't the case for Native people. Beginning in 1860, the federal government provided for the establishment of 357 boarding schools for Native Americans in twenty-nine states. Many were operated by Christian churches.

Abuse, starvation, disease, and death haunted these institutions throughout the nineteenth and early twentieth centuries. I spoke to K. Tsianina Lomawaima, the daughter of a Mvskoke/Creek Nation boarding school survivor, who is a retired university professor and the author of three acclaimed books about the Native American educational experience. Her research explores how boarding schools were designed to destroy Native sovereignty by breaking the chain of cultural transmission. "That's not a policy that was motivated by, 'How do we best care for these children?' Care was totally tangential. [The motivation was:] How do we continue the process of dispossessing Native people from their lands?" In words applied by journalist Adam Serwer to President Trump's family separation policy: the cruelty is the point.

This is why academic and advocate Laura Briggs calls "child taking" a form of terrorism.

The boarding schools were succeeded and complemented by federal policies that promoted the adoption of Native children by white families. One report found as many as one-third of Native children were separated from their families and communities between 1941 and 1967.

Native activists lobbied for the Indian Child Welfare Act (ICWA), passed in 1978, as a counterweight. In some ways this law is considered model legislation for preserving families. It promotes children being placed with kin and tribe whenever possible.

But Native children are still being removed from their families at a higher rate than any other racial or ethnic group in the United States. A 2014 study found about 15 percent of Native children and 11 percent of Black children could expect to enter foster care before their eighteenth birthday. The rate for white children is just 5 percent. As this book went to press, the ICWA faced a challenge at the Supreme Court, brought by a white Evangelical couple who had some trouble adopting the Cherokee and Navajo boy they had fostered.

ORPHAN TRAINS

For urban immigrant families on the East Coast, child removal took yet a different form in the nineteenth century.

Charles Loring Brace studied at Yale Divinity School and was ordained as a Congregationalist minister in 1849. While more carefree youths spent their Grand Tours of Europe at the opera or in fashionable drawing rooms, he toured European prisons. Back in

New York City, he worked at the Five Points Mission in the city's most notorious slum. He became obsessed with the swelling ranks of poor children, particularly children of Irish and German immigrants, whom he referred to as "street rats."

"The intensity of the American temperament is felt in every fibre of these children of poverty and vice. Their crimes have the unrestrained and sanguinary character of a race accustomed to overcome all obstacles," he wrote, spinning a portrait of innate hyper-criminality that recalls the "super-predator" myth wielded against Black youth in the 1990s. "Thousands are the children of poor foreigners, who have permitted them to grow up without school, education, or religion.... At length, a great multitude of ignorant, untrained, passionate, irreligious boys and young men are formed, who become the 'dangerous class' of our city."

Brace's solution was chilling: a transport train that would take children to live with, and toil for, strangers on farms across the country. As Brace's organization proudly stated in its first annual report, "We have thus far sent off to homes in the country, or to places where they could earn an honest living, 164 boys and 43 girls, of whom some 20 were taken from prison, where they had been placed for being homeless on the streets."

Most of these Orphan Train riders were not orphans. "The great majority were the children of poor or degraded people, who were leaving them to grow up neglected in the streets. They were found by our visitors at the turning point of their lives, and sent to friendly homes, where they would be removed from the overwhelming temptations which poverty and neglect certainly occasion in a great city."

On arrival in a new town, children were lined up on the stage of the local opera house or town hall and given away to strangers. Siblings could be split up. Brace boasted this practice would improve lives, remove a "poisonous influence" from the city, and save the public money. The Orphan Trains and the "mercy trains," carrying babies acquired by the New York Foundling Hospital, removed an estimated 150,000–200,000 children from the only homes they'd ever known between 1854 and 1930. Well into the 1990s, some survivors of the Orphan Trains testified to a "nightmare" of physical, sexual, and psychological abuse.

Brace is honored as a humanitarian to this day. He founded the New York Children's Aid Society, which today takes in over $125 million in revenue each year. Its website calls the Orphan Trains "an ambitious and controversial social experiment that is now recognized as the beginning of the foster care system in the United States."

With such beginnings, how much has the system progressed?

THE TURN AWAY

Our government has never stopped disproportionately removing immigrant, Black, and Brown children and those living in poverty from their homes. But for the past half century, the national emphasis on policing families rather than helping them hasn't rested on a rhetoric of explicit racism and dehumanization. We don't call children "rats" anymore or talk about the need to "civilize" them. Instead we have intensified the demonization of parents, with successive waves of moral panic about the prevalence of child abuse.

THE BONES TELL A STORY

This emphasis comes in part from the crusade of a doctor named Henry Kempe. He fled the Nazis alone as a teenager. When he was training as a pediatric radiologist, X-ray imaging was becoming more sophisticated. The technology held a powerful mystique in that postwar era. Superman has X-ray vision; so did the "man with the X-ray eyes," in a 1963 sci-fi classic. Kempe argued in a 1962 journal article that X-rays could, and often did, reveal repeated injuries to children over time: "To the informed physician, the bones tell a story the child is too young or too frightened to tell."

The article, "The Battered Child Syndrome," created a sensation. It intimated a hidden epidemic of physical abuse that expert doctors could discover. Even if parents lied and denied, as they were expected to, Kempe argued that doctors had a duty to report their suspicions. He told a newspaper in 1970, "We think far too much of the 'rights' of the parents and not enough of the 'rights' of the child."

Today's critics of the child welfare system agree with that sentiment. They agree with Kempe, too, that child abuse is serious, prevalent, and often hidden. The more material advantages a family has, the more likely it is to remain hidden. The attorney in California who spoke to me on background said that any time a white parent shows up in child welfare proceedings, she steels herself for a horrific tale of abuse. Things have to get very bad in a relatively privileged family to come to the attention of the authorities.

"Child physical abuse and sexual abuse is a real problem. It's terrible and it needs to be addressed. I never want to be portrayed as pro–child abuse," Mical Raz says. Raz is a physician and professor of history and health policy at the University of Rochester. In her 2020 book *Abusive Policies: How the American Child Welfare System Lost Its Way*, Raz focuses on the 1960s and early 1970s.

Kempe revealed the reality of serious physical abuse of children at a time when corporal punishment was still widespread at home and at schools and domestic violence against women barely recognized. And he lobbied hard. By the late 1960s, forty-nine states had laws mandating the report of suspected child abuse.

As a doctor, Kempe naturally promoted a clinical model for the prevention of child abuse. He focused on raising public awareness, and early detection in a clinical setting. But unlike, say, rickets or appendicitis, there was no easy prevention or prescription that didn't involve a lot of public spending.

PARENTS ANONYMOUS

Around the same time Kempe's work was causing a sensation in medical circles, in the late 1960s, a woman known as Jolly K. went to a psychiatric social worker named Leonard Lieber for help to stop abusing her young daughter, Faith. The two of them founded an organization called Parents Anonymous, a system of support groups for abusive parents, modeled on other types of recovery programs. Most of its members, like Jolly K., were relatively well-off white women, a reflection of who was likely to have time to access mental health programs or felt comfortable doing so.

Raz's book states that Parents Anonymous, which still exists today, may have been helpful for many parents. But its messaging conflated all forms of abuse, creating moral equivalency among yelling at children, ignoring them, and beating and sexually molesting them. And their "recovery" model focused on individual psychological motivations for child abuse, rather than structural issues like the stresses of poverty.

Parents Anonymous gained national attention when Jolly K. testified, emotionally, in support of a new piece of legislation sponsored by Senator Walter Mondale. The bill, the Child Abuse Prevention and Treatment Act, or CAPTA, established a federal mandate to report abuse. Mondale was invested in showing that child abuse cut across social classes. This, he believed, would broaden his bill's popularity. Jolly K.'s testimony made that point for him.

CAPTA passed in 1973. Recall from Chapter 3 that Senator Mondale sponsored the Comprehensive Child Development Act to create a federally subsidized daycare system. President Richard Nixon vetoed that bill in 1971. CAPTA, a regulatory mandate without a serious spending commitment, fared better.

Instead of getting an expanded public program to help support their children, American families would get an expanded policing apparatus to punish them for failing to support their children.

By 1978, twenty states had adopted universal mandatory requirements for any adult to report any suspicion of any kind of abuse of any child. The emphasis on early detection comes from Kempe's public health model of prevention. But there was never as much emphasis on "treating" or preventing child abuse as there was on reporting it. In fact, as Raz has documented, one often drove out the other.

"Florida was the first state to implement a child abuse reporting hot-line," she wrote. "In 1971, the state began publicizing a hotline—toll-free and open twenty-four hours a day, seven days a week—and the number of reports increased from just 17 in 1970 to 19,120 the following year. Yet state politicians made no funding appropriations to deal with this increase in reports."

FIRE ALARMS WITHOUT FIRE ENGINES

In other words, we installed fire alarms in every school, camp, and doctor's office but didn't pay for fire engines or sprinkler systems. Addressing child maltreatment requires a whole society: income supports, family counseling, substance abuse treatment. The United States didn't substantially create that. Instead we extended a centuries-long practice of overseeing, judging, and punishing low-income families and families of color under a new justification.

Raz trained as a physician. She saw how mandatory reporting went awry specifically in hospitals. "If you call Child Protective Services on anything you don't like, essentially it becomes our way of policing family behavior. You know, we say, well, we'll call CPS on you if you don't come back for your next appointment. Or, this kid has bad teeth, let's call CPS for dental care." This is a fallacy, she says. "We know that most investigations actually don't end with a provision of services."

There may be situations—like custody disputes, family or neighbors feuding, or landlords who want a new tenant—where CPS is called simply because someone wants an upper hand. In other cases, people really want to help. "There's the fantasy that this is helpful. But the reality is, it's not experienced as helpful for parents and very, very rarely is it actually helpful."

The urge to rescue children is visceral, overwhelming. But child welfare as it exists violates the principle of "first, do no harm." Being removed from your home, no matter the reason, is inherently traumatic. The instability of foster care is its own trauma. The national target for "stability" is averaging one and a half foster placements each year, which many states do not meet. Some children, especially older children and those with behavioral problems, are moved dozens of times, making it impossible for them to form secure attachments. And independent studies suggest around one in three children experience some form of abuse while in foster care, including by foster siblings who are often traumatized themselves.

KHAMLA AND JONAH

During the months he spent with Maya, Robert, and Jonah, Khamla did well in remote school. He was as calm as Jonah was explosive and often seemed to be able to calm down his friend with a gentle touch. They loved to play the video game *Rocket League* together on their handheld Nintendo Switches, build with Legos, and carry Teddy the cat from room to room. They rode scooters together, Khamla always a little more cautious than Jonah. When he stumbled, he would hang his head and his choppy bangs would fall into his face.

He also felt sad, worried, responsible for his mother, and eager to live with her again. Maya and Robert made sure that he could visit her, in person, once a week with COVID protocols in place; she called him on his own private smartphone almost every day. He had been her translator and her main conduit to the outside world almost since they arrived in the United States. This dynamic, common in immigrant families, is sometimes called "parentification." Young people tasked with these roles can end up with more self-efficacy but also feelings of exhaustion and loneliness.

In early visits, she would tell him that she hadn't eaten and was too scared to go food shopping. Eventually, she started doing better and would send Khamla back to Maya and Robert with bags of durian candy for him and Jonah.

Maya believes that Khamla's parents and other family put pressure on him to suppress the situation at home, but Khamla somehow found the courage to tell the truth instead and ask for help.

Later on, he stopped talking about how his mother was doing or how the visits were going. Maya felt like he didn't want to get her in trouble. "'She's good,' he told me about his mother. How do you feel after you see her? 'I'm OK.'"

Maya and Robert were negotiating their place in this young boy's life. "I don't want to overstep," Maya told me. "I don't totally feel like I'm parenting. I feel like I'm just trying to be a support person. Khamla has a mom. We're just doing what we can do to get along well and to provide stability.... On the other hand it does also feel like parenting. It's confusing."

PUNISHING POOR FAMILIES AND CHILD WELFARE ABOLITION

In June 2021, the legal scholar Dorothy Roberts gave a remote keynote address at a symposium at Columbia University. Her 1999 book *Shattered Bonds: The Color of Child Welfare* is considered the foundation text for the movement now called child welfare abolition. "If you came with no preconceptions about the purpose of the child welfare system," she said in her speech, "you would have to conclude that it's an institution designed to monitor, regulate, and punish poor Black families."

Roberts noted that since the book's publication she'd been involved in many years of failed reform efforts. Many cities are under court order to reform their child welfare systems. Yet racial disparities in child welfare are as bad as they've ever been or worse. The symposium, called "Strengthened Bonds," was organized to honor and amplify her book after two decades in which little has changed.

Family separation at the border, and the treatment of unaccompanied minors, became a national scandal under President Trump.

Family separation by the child welfare system is different. Its violations go unnoticed to people whose lives are never touched by a call from CPS.

Every few years the horrific, heart-wrenching murder of a child by his or her abusive family member makes headlines. And the response is a call for child welfare to crack down. But like "tough on crime" policies, "tough on parent" policies don't tend to make enforcement more effective, and they don't address prevention. They burden child welfare systems with more investigative responsibilities and burden families with more scrutiny.

Racism, two centuries of maternalist politics dividing mothers into deserving and undeserving, and a moral panic over child abuse that dates back half a century. Take it all together, and privileged people are ready to believe that only irredeemable mothers are in danger of losing their children.

Maya, an educated white parent, had no qualms telling me, a journalist, that she had fits of rage when Jonah's behavior got over-the-top frustrating. For several years she had been a single mom getting regular calls about her son's behavior from San Francisco Public Schools, including for violent outbursts, and she barely knew what it meant to call CPS. When she did come into contact with CPS, it was them asking her to take in someone else's child.

I do not presume to judge her. Their home, when I visited, was clearly full of love. She and Robert were by all appearances scrupulously conscientious parents to both Khamla and Jonah. But the double standard is obvious. Some families fear a knock at the door, and some don't.

In her 2021 speech, Roberts said that now might finally be the moment for change. The Movement for Black Lives has brought once-radical ideas closer to the political mainstream, like funding social services instead of police, closing jails, and eliminating cash bail. Nonprofits like Brooklyn Family Defense Project are providing families with consistent and skilled legal representation in child welfare cases. Advocates want to end the practice of removal for poverty alone, to place more children with kin or family friends, and to eliminate group homes.

A FOSTER CHILD GROWN UP

Roberts raised one more reason for hope of reshaping the archipelago, maybe the most important reason. The people directly affected by the foster system are increasingly sharing their experiences. One of those children grew up to be Patricia Stamper, the mother I spent time with in DC.

Patricia was born in Oakland, California. As she later learned, her mother was intellectually disabled and gave up her rights to her daughter before she left the maternity ward.

A woman who volunteered at her mother's adult day program took baby Patricia in. When Patricia was around three or four years old, as she recalls, she was home with chicken pox. Her foster mother, a mail carrier, came home from work and walked in on her husband molesting Patricia. An older woman, she suffered a heart attack and stroke more or less on the spot. Her foster mother's extended family, who belonged to the Seventh-Day Adventist Church, came on the scene and moved her to Compton, in Los Angeles.

The early days are hazy. Patricia remembers a group home where she would hide in the laundry room to read at night after lights-out. She also remembers a meeting being called where a family told her they would keep her as a long-term foster placement rather than pursue adoption. She says she must have been in kindergarten, because it was during the Rodney King riots in Los Angeles in 1992, and school was ordered closed. "They had a meeting to discuss me. They thought it would be in my best interest to keep the case open so I can get as much benefits as possible. And it would help [my foster mother] financially too. She got money to keep me, and she used that money to pay to send me to private school."

Patricia got good grades and was an athlete and a debutante. She spent her spare time volunteering for church fundraisers, which ingrained a lifelong habit of community service. She remembers an elderly lady in the church handing over her car keys so Patricia could learn to drive. "I was blown away by that."

On the one hand, she felt cared for by the whole community; on the other hand, she never felt like she fully belonged to anyone in particular. "'This is my *other* daughter.' Like, I was always introduced like that. I didn't like that. One day I was like, the other daughter, what do you mean by that? I felt like I was always tolerated but not really wanted."

Her family asked whether she wanted to change her last name to theirs, but she kept her birth name so that her mother could find her.

Patricia remembers the exact date she left California for Washington, DC, for college. "It's August 20, 2004, when I landed at BWI."

She never stopped trying to find her mother. Around 2005—she remembers it was when PDFs became searchable on Google—she spotted her mother's name in what turned out to be a newsletter for the adult day program she was in. She called them up, verified who she was, and flew out to California to meet her mother. She was twenty-three years old.

Her mother didn't seem to understand who she was. "She told me, 'I have a baby. This baby has so much hair. Her name is Patricia.' And I explained to her, 'I'm your baby. I grew up.' And she kept looking at me. And I showed her the youngest picture that I have of myself. I think I was like four or five, it was the day I came from Palo Alto to Compton. And I have nothing younger than that." Patricia's mother was moved to a different institution, and in July 2020 she finally tracked her down again. After the pandemic, she hopes to go out and see her again, maybe bring the boys.

7 MOTHERS AND OTHERS

OPEN THE SCHOOLS!!!

—Trump, Twitter, August 4, 2020

If you look at children, children are almost—and I would almost say definitely—but almost immune from this disease.

—Trump, *Fox and Friends*, August 5, 2020

August 6, 2020, US death toll passes 160,000

August 16, 2020, US death toll passes 170,000

Washington, DC, public schools started the year remotely on August 31, 2020. The first time I ever spoke to Patricia Stamper on the phone was a few days later, for a story for NPR. Pete, her husband, was out at work. Patrick, nineteen months old, was finally down for his nap. I ask about the noise in the background.

"You're on my virtual meet and greet," Patricia said, for one of the two classrooms she was supporting as a special education aide. "Hold on."

"Would another time be better?"

"No, no, you're good. You're good. It's just—I'm in between meetings. One meeting is running over. My son brought me the phone, he's like, 'Mommy! Mommy! Your phone! Your 11:30!'"

That was PJ. The day before, the second day of kindergarten, PJ had carried the laptop into his bedroom and started showing off his toys to his classmates. "He was like, I'm bored. I want to be like Ryan"—a child YouTube star with thirty million followers—Patricia explained. He had everyone's attention pretty quickly. "He's smart, but he's mischievous," said Patricia. "He's a Leo."

Other parents started texting Patricia. The teacher asked for a conference. "And I'm like, first of all, you do realize you're asking a five-year-old to sit in front of a screen for three to four hours at a time. And it is hard to check him. I'm trying to do my job and, you know, bounce back and forth, but I'm only one person."

THE PRIMAL SCREAM

This chapter is about the ordinary and daily disaster of being a primary caregiver in 2020.

While a lot of this chapter deals with working, partnered mothers, I do my best to take in the experiences of other primary caregivers. Like Shirley Leake, in Jackson, Mississippi, eighty-five years old and raising the twelve-year-old child of a relative on her own. Like Kirk Gallegos, who works construction and has sole custody of his three daughters in Barstow, California. Like my close friend Gia Kagan-Trenchard, in Brooklyn, New York, who came out as a trans woman during the pandemic and quit her job to take care of two elementary-school-aged children, while her wife continued to work long hours as a health-care executive.

Most of the social science research that I'll rely on in this chapter, not to mention much of the history, is biased toward the cisgender, heterosexual norm. Those are limited views of the world. Families are a lot more complicated than that.

One in four children in the United States is living in a single-parent household, the highest percentage in the world. In five out of six cases, that parent is the mother.

That does mean 3.25 million children live with only their father. And grandparents, 2.7 million of them, are raising their grandchildren—a number that's risen in some places over the past decade because of the opioid crisis.

There's an estimated 114,000 same-sex couples raising children in this country. Trans and gender-nonconforming parents and caregivers have distinct experiences as well, though there isn't much research about them. More and more people each year feel comfortable telling pollsters about their gender identity, so estimates of the size of the trans and gender-nonconforming population keep rising. And in June 2020, the city of Somerville, Massachusetts, became the first in the country to pass an ordinance conferring the legal rights of marriage on polyamorous domestic groups.

Many researchers are intrigued by the prospect that families outside the patriarchal and nuclear norms might be doing things better. For example, some research suggests that same-sex couples tend to divide domestic labor more equally, reducing household conflict. A small survey from Australia done in the early days of the pandemic found that single mothers and same-sex dads were less stressed than heterosexual parents. (Lesbian mothers were a mixed bag.) Single mothers, in particular, reported less work-life balance conflict; they may have had less help, but at least they didn't have to fight over who was unloading the dishwasher.

MONEY RUNS OUT IN AUGUST

A few new miseries struck in August and September. Number one, the CARES Act expired at the end of July. The $600-a-week federal supplement for unemployment benefits that had been there since April? Gone.

Phil Fisher at the University of Oregon, who had been surveying families with young children each month, saw a dramatic change from July to August.

"In July, when we surveyed families, we found 20 percent of all households with children under age five reporting that they were having trouble paying for at least one basic need," like housing, food, or transportation.

"In August, we found that the rates of material hardship in this age group of children had gone up to 40 percent." Doubled in one month.

And just after those federal benefits ran out, there was a large bump in mothers leaving the workforce.

"In September, 865,000 women left the workforce," C. Nicole Mason told me—four times as many women as men left in the identical time period. She is CEO of the Institute for Women's Policy Research.

To clarify: There is a difference between losing your job and exiting the workforce. If you lose your job, you are unemployed and presumed to be seeking work. Leaving the workforce means you are not looking for work. You disappear from the unemployment rolls.

"People ask me why" so many women were leaving at that moment, Mason continued. After all, there were different levels of lockdowns and restrictions around the country, but August was a comparative low point for COVID cases in the United States, and hiring was up overall.

"I was like, oh, well, it's kind of a no-brainer. That's when schools were supposed to open and they didn't. And so families had to make some tough choices."

The patchwork that was school reopening is the subject of the next chapter. For our purposes here, let's note that school buildings reopened full-time in only a few places in the fall of 2020. The start of the school year was also delayed, sometimes multiple times, adding to the uncertainty.

It was mostly moms who bore the brunt of those choices. One paper, looking at families with elementary-school-aged students, showed a strong relationship between school reopening status in the fall of 2020 and levels of mothers', but not fathers', employment. An increase of one day per week of in-person schooling was associated with a nearly one-percentage-point increase in mothers in the workforce.

Mason noted that the lack of childcare could be ruinous for single mothers in particular. This is a direct consequence of the family policing we talked about in the previous chapter. "For many women, the only viable choice was to exit. It wasn't about like, oh, I have another spouse to shoulder the burden. [It's] I could be arrested if my children are home alone."

It happened, she told me, to Shaina Bell in Liberty Township, Ohio. She was arrested in February 2021. Her offense was leaving two of her children alone while she went to her job at a Little Caesar's. They were staying in a Motel 6 because they didn't have permanent housing. The older child was ten years old. Bell was just twenty-four, and Black— which is significant because, as outlined in Chapter 6, fully half of Black children are investigated by the state before they turn eighteen.

UNEVEN AND STALLED

It shocked me to learn that women have made essentially no progress in labor force participation in the twenty-first century. We hit the peak of six in ten women working all the way back in 1999. That year the R&B girl group TLC topped the charts with "No Scrubs," about an independent woman rejecting an unemployed man.

Sociologist Paula England called it in the 2010 paper "The Gender Revolution: Uneven and Stalled": "Because the devaluation of activities done by women has changed little, women have had strong incentive to enter male jobs, but men have had little incentive to take on female activities or jobs."

At the same time women were joining the workforce, from the 1960s onward, men have been leaving the workforce, partly because the population has been aging. So in January 2020, with unemployment at a fifty-year low, women crossed over 50 percent of the paid workforce. This was hailed as a milestone and a sign of greatly equal things to come.

Then lockdowns put the economy into a medically induced coma. Women lost just over half of the jobs that vanished in March and April 2020, the first recession in US history where women lost most of the jobs.

Pandemic lockdowns cut retail, food service, hospitality, and childcare. Black and Latina women without a college degree lost more jobs than others. It was dubbed a "she-cession." It stood in contrast to the Great Recession in 2008. That was a housing bust, which eliminated a lot of construction jobs, which meant it was deemed a "he-cession."

One in ten working mothers with children under eighteen said they quit a job because of COVID. Half specifically cited school closures. One in three working-age women who were out of work blamed a lack of childcare. Only 12 percent of men said the same.

MOST MOTHERS KEPT WORKING

Most of the mothers I'm following in this book stayed attached to the labor force. Mothers are actually more likely to work than women in general.

Heather got laid off from her job as a home health aide at the beginning of the pandemic and then from her job at a homeless shelter after her son was injured and her childcare arrangements weren't working. She pressed on, trying to raise money to start her own nonprofit aiding the homeless.

Patricia Stamper kept working remotely for the DC public schools and, when she could, as a delivery driver for DoorDash and as a referee for local sports games. Jeannie kept teaching in person in Oklahoma and taking portrait photos on the side. Maya kept working for a community foundation in San Francisco. She was technically eligible for twelve weeks of leave twice over, both to care for her mother with cancer and to ease the transition of taking Khamla on as a foster child. But she'd been laid off a decade earlier, during the Great Recession, as a single parent. She didn't want to put her career at risk at the age of almost fifty. "I think it would have felt too insecure to not work when there were so many people who were becoming unemployed." She also found some positives in continuing to work. "Considering everything, I feel like I got some really big things accomplished, and it felt good to be able to continue to sort of be of service during that time," she says.

Dara Kass worked even harder than before. Starting from when she wrote about her own bout of COVID in March, she was asked to comment publicly and advise people privately on the course of the pandemic. She appeared on television and published popular press articles while also treating patients. She never seriously considered stepping back. "Part of the benefit of being in the pandemic, and living in New York, I've been able to identify something I can do that's a part of the solution, even when things are really, really bad," she explains.

> When I got infected, I could be public about that. Public-facing communication helped me compartmentalize the anxiety about having it. Then when I recovered, I was able to track my own antibodies and I was able to publicize that.
>
> I am making a very, very meaningful difference in people's lives at a time when they are scared. And that's a gift. Not everybody gets to do that, especially in the pandemic when everyone is feeling isolated and afraid and lost. I've had a purpose. So why would I want to give it away? Why would I want to walk away from that?

None of these mothers took pandemic caregiver leave. In March 2020 Congress passed a new law providing twelve weeks of paid leave, capped at $200 per day, specifically for employees whose children's schools or daycares had closed. But there were carve-outs—for large companies, for small companies, for health care and emergency responders—that excluded almost half of private-sector workers. In the end, the biggest legacy of that law may be the dozens of employment lawsuits filed, mostly by mothers, who were fired when they asked their bosses to take this leave or for some other concession to the burdens of caregiving.

The sheer obliviousness of employers during this crisis might be best symbolized by what happened to Buffy Wicks. In August 2020 the California assembly member was denied a proxy vote, an option offered to some of her colleagues who were deemed at high risk of COVID-19. So she showed up in person on the legislative floor—with her one-month-old daughter Elly in her arms—and cast a deciding yes vote on a California bill to expand paid leave. "It's either ironic or serendipitous," she told MSNBC. "Had I not been there, it potentially wouldn't have passed."

EVERYTHING GOT HARDER

Mothers kept working for wages if they possibly could. It was just that everything got harder. The loss of full-time childcare and the need to homeschool were both associated with an increased risk of unemployment, reduced hours, and other negative economic outcomes for mothers—but not for fathers. Almost half of working mothers said they took unpaid sick leave when their child's school or daycare was closed owing to COVID. A study based on census data found mothers with young children reduced their work hours four to five times more than fathers did at the outset of the pandemic. They may not have lost jobs, but they lost income and professional status.

Speaking personally, I worked harder than I ever had before during the pandemic. There was a huge appetite suddenly for stories about education. I went from filing stories once a week to three times a week, while also working on this book. Like Dara, I felt a stronger sense of purpose and commitment to my work and wouldn't have wanted to take time off.

At the start of lockdown we had a three-year-old who needed near-constant supervision. My third grader, in public school, generally had about an hour's worth of unchallenging remote lessons per day. We were grateful that our downstairs tenant, who lives alone and is a freelancer, agreed to share a bubble with us and provide twenty hours a week of childcare in exchange for a break on rent.

My husband works a very challenging job and makes much more money than I do. But he tries hard to be egalitarian. During lockdown, we divided up the direct hours of daily childcare as equally as possible. But there were subtle imbalances common to many straight couples. For example, he had set up his home office, years before COVID, in the basement. That meant he was literally insulated from the sounds of unhappy children. I had a small office upstairs, next to the kids' bedroom. No matter who was supposed to be in charge, my preschooler rattled the door regularly or just stormed in if I forgot to lock it, sometimes asking for a quick hug, sometimes in full meltdown. I know her voice came through live on air at least once.

Most of all, I felt burdened with a new mental load. Before COVID, I managed the schedules and planned the activities. I write about schools for a living, which at least provided some justification for the fact that I was the one to research preschools and after-school programs and summer camps, to make spreadsheets and show up to parent-teacher conferences and PTA meetings. I also did the grocery shopping and meal planning and most of the cooking.

My husband picked up relaxing, fully optional household tasks during the pandemic, perfecting his sourdough bread and kombucha. I got dinner on the table night after night, subscribed to several new grocery delivery services, and sweated over inventory management of our new stockpiles of marinara sauce and dried beans. Once I had a full-on breakdown because we were out of dark green vegetables and running to the grocery store for a single item seemed at the time like an out-of-bounds risk.

MOMS WORRIED MORE ABOUT COVID ITSELF

As my kale freak-out illustrates, the fact that this was a *public health* crisis hit moms especially hard. Of the many papers I read in preparation for this chapter, one that really stuck with me was titled "Dad, Wash Your Hands." The paper, by Janani Umamaheswar and Catherine Tan, found, based on interviews, that "gender differences in attitudes toward risk are influenced by the unique and strenuous care work responsibilities generated by the COVID-19 pandemic, which are borne primarily by women—and from which men are exempt."

Gender differences showed up in many ways in the response to the pandemic. Men were more likely to get COVID. They were less likely to wear masks. When the vaccine appeared they were slower to get it.

There is a lot of background research that predicts that women would respond more strongly to a public health emergency. We are generally more aware of risk than men are. We worry more, especially about threats to our families. We pay more attention to health in particular. We are overrepresented in health care as well as other caring professions. We are twice as likely to visit the doctor for preventative care and annual checkups.

Mothers in general also already tend to oversee family health through grocery shopping, meal planning and cooking, tending to colds and booboos, purchasing sunscreen in the summer and boots in the winter, laundry, cleaning.

Pandemics are social predators, spreading through close contact with other people. Women have a clearer picture of friendship and kinship networks. We are socialized to focus more on how our decisions affect other people. We also feel more responsible for the well-being of the people in our network. So women, as a group, are more concerned not only about their own health but also about the health of others close to them.

In short, women tended to be more worried about coronavirus. They did more of the work to keep everyone safe. That contributed, in a vicious cycle, to their being more worried, as well as more tired. Men were more likely to be exempted from all of the above.

COVID AND THE MENTAL LOAD

COVID was constant risk recalculation, backup plans, emotional labor, fear, uncertainty, and doubt.

Do I send the kids to school or daycare or keep them home? Do I order takeout? Wipe down my groceries? Is it OK to see Grandma with masks on? Are my friends on the group text mad at me? Is my daughter just in a mood or is she depressed? Is that tickle in the back of my throat COVID? Do I trust the CDC or the president or my friends on Facebook?

Each of these questions could prompt what Dara called her "rabbit holes." "I constantly accumulate and aggregate that information in my mind"—not only for herself and her family but for her broader community—"and then basically amplify that on social media, because I don't know what else to do with a void of leadership and messaging."

Not only was she solving problems and gaming things out for her own family; she started getting texts and emails at all hours from friends and friends of friends and total strangers, most often moms, who needed COVID advice about quarantine and exposure and activities and travel and testing and on and on. "People ask me to make the decisions they don't want to make."

Dara's husband, Michael, was, at times, the naysayer. "He thinks I'm a doomsday person for a lot of this stuff, but then when it comes to fruition, he says, 'oh, you're right.'"

MY HUSBAND THINKS I'M CRAZY

Jess Calarco, a sociologist at Indiana University, was already doing qualitative research, interviewing mothers about their well-being, when the pandemic hit. She pivoted to asking them about their pandemic experiences. "Back in March, the moms are telling us how they were staying up until midnight or waking up at 5:00 a.m. to be able to get their work done and then care for their kids and be the teachers during the day."

She said the mothers who kept doing all the things—like her and me—worried her the most. "I am especially worried about the women who are still employed and also still have their kids at home without childcare, without school. I think those moms are going to be hurt in their careers, because it's often hard to do the level of work that they'll need to get the promotions and to get the raises and maintain on track in their careers. And they're also getting slammed in terms of their mental health, in terms of their relationships, in terms of their ability to remain patient with their partners and their kids."

In a paper with the pointed title "My Husband Thinks I'm Crazy," Calarco found four in ten of her subjects, mothers with young children, were more frustrated with their partners during the pandemic. This was especially true when the fathers didn't help as much with caregiving and when they were dismissive of their concerns about coronavirus.

And here's the kicker: Who did mothers blame for all of this? Not their partners. "Mothers blame themselves for these conflicts," Calarco found, "and feel responsible for reducing them, including by leaving the workforce, beginning use of antidepressants, or ignoring their own concerns about COVID-19."

WHAT DADS DID

Are you a cisgender, heterosexual dad reading this chapter who thinks things were pretty evenly split at your house? Years of polling, including during the pandemic, suggest that your partner doesn't agree with you. Do you think you might actually do more of the direct parenting or bear more of the mental load regarding the children? Well, maybe your wife is one of the 3 percent of mothers who thinks so too. Ask her.

It's not that fathers didn't help—but to quote Sonya Michel, the historian of childcare from Chapter 3, "notice how I used that word, *helping*." Most studies found that fathers who were able to work from home did pick up more domestic work, especially early on. Some surveys found that men did more childcare but not necessarily more housework. Others found that changes in the beginning didn't hold up for long, with men and women slipping back into more gendered roles within a few months. Women did more of the remote schooling in particular, especially among couples at higher income levels.

Daniel Carlson, a sociologist at the University of Utah, explains:

The division of work has become more equal. But at the same time, women are doing more than men. And I know that that sounds like, how is that possible? But if you think about it in terms of what men were doing before, even a marginal increase in their labor is going to result in more equality.

So if you had, like, a couple that was doing twenty hours of housework total before the pandemic and the female partner is doing fifteen hours and the male partner was doing five hours, he's doing a quarter of the housework. Right. Let's say that he increases his amount of labor, you know, by five hours and hers goes up by eight. He's now doing a much larger proportion of the housework, over 30 percent.

The man is doing ten hours a week; the woman is now doing twenty-three. "So, it's gotten more equal, even as the gap between men and women has grown."

The math is confusing. And this is how fights ignite: a husband may focus on how much he's stepped up, while the wife sees only how she's doing even more than before.

These inequities held true for most of the mothers I spent time with.

Jeannie's ex George was working long hours out of the home, often six days a week, at a chicken feed mill. He was living in the house, but they typically communicated by text. He was a safe person to leave the kids with, and he helped financially. But she despaired of getting him to make dinner, oversee schooling, do the grocery shopping, pick up the house, take care of the pets, or drive the girls back and forth to gymnastics, more than an hour each way. "He was supposed to step up. I told him, I said...you're going to have to help me. I cannot do it all. And he said OK. And he did not. I don't think he knows how."

George was pretty forthcoming about this. "She definitely was overwhelmed. I didn't help her as much as I should. And we got into several arguments about that. She was calling my job an escape so I didn't have to help."

Patricia's husband, Pete, was hands on with his kids when he was around. But like George he also worked more hours out of the house than Patricia. She did most of the cooking and cleaning.

There is some research indicating that when women earn more than their husbands, as Patricia does, they actually do *even more* of the domestic labor. And even when husbands are unemployed and wives are working, on average the women still are doing more at home. As sociologist Aliya Rao documents in her June 2020 book *Crunch Time: How Married Couples Confront Unemployment*, both husband and wife protect the man's time and his ego so he can look for a new job. If a mother becomes unemployed, by contrast, she is more likely to take on more housework and care work than ever and redefine herself as a stay-at-home mom. This leads in turn to longer periods of unemployment.

With the possible exception of Pete, Robert was the most highly involved father among the families I talked to. Maybe this is related to the fact that he is an avowed feminist, and both he and Maya had moved in queer circles for years. And the couple, if anything, became more egalitarian during the pandemic.

When the pandemic started, Robert and Maya were engaged and had been living together for five years. But they didn't fully think of Robert as Jonah's dad or stepdad. Robert had joint custody of his older son, Rust, from a previous relationship, and they parented in parallel: "Jonah is my kid, Rust is Robert's kid," as Maya put it. Managing Jonah's life involved coordinating with a whole team of professionals and frequent meetings with the school, and that fell to Maya.

That dynamic continued through the spring of 2020. Gradually, they worked out a more equal tradeoff of time during the day. Still, it took time for Maya to trust Robert to follow Jonah's care plan and routines. She believed in the importance of order and ritual, printed schedules and timers. He was gentle by nature and more inclined to let things like bedtime slide.

Things changed again when Khamla moved in. With Khamla, Robert and Maya felt in a funny way like they were equal coparents for the first time. "Rust and I didn't do well together, Jonah and Rust didn't do well together, Robert and I didn't do well dealing with Rust together. It's just been very challenging," said Maya. "So it's been great to have Khamla here. It's kind of like a fresh start. We're on even ground with him."

Dara Kass was working shifts at the hospital while her husband, Michael, worked from home. They had full-time, live-in help from their au pair, plus occasional help from her parents. But she clearly took on more of the mental load, including the decision making about activities, everyone's health, and remote learning.

Dara said her husband did step up. She gave him a lot of credit for buying the family's Hanukkah gifts for the first time ever in their fifteen-year marriage. "It's amazing. It's amazing. It's amazing. It's amazing. And it's not that he wouldn't have before. It's like, when is he ever home to get the packages and when is he ever home to wrap the presents and when is he ever home to make the list and double-check it?"

Dara, let's remember, is an emergency room doctor. I asked her, When are you ever home to do those things? "Yes, we're both [normally] working out of the house. But women historically were the ones paying attention to everything."

DEEP PATRIARCHAL NORMS

Whether or not they are breadwinners, sometimes women who are powerful and accomplished at work feel the need to take the lioness's share of care and oversight of their children at home. Psychologists sometimes call this "maternal gatekeeping" or "perfectionism," but that sounds like victim blaming to me. I agree more with Jess Calarco: "There are these deep patriarchal norms that exist in society and they tell women, oftentimes for the economic benefit and power of men, that they should be the ones who are devoting their whole selves to their children and to family."

Some sociologists call this behavior "gender display" (like a peacock) or even, intriguingly, "neutralizing gender deviance"—bringing home the bacon and frying it up in a pan and also washing that pan and also putting the kids to bed and doing the laundry, all so my husband feels better about himself and I feel more like a real woman. My friend Emily calls it "momchismo."

These patriarchal norms may be most policed by other women. Starting in the second half of the twentieth century, women, especially privileged women with education and earning potential, felt the need to justify their choice to continue to occupy a traditional role in a world of broader opportunities. So they changed their job description from "housewife" to "stay-at-home mom," putting the emphasis on the children. They basically went pro as moms. Scholars dubbed the approach "intensive mothering" (with an emphasis on the emotional investment) or "concerted cultivation" (emphasizing the time and money that goes to scheduling and enrichment). The media called it "helicopter parenting" (blaming moms for being neurotic).

All of this is presented as what's best for children. So women who work outside the house feel pressure to meet the new, impossible standard. That's how you get this paradox where mothers are actually spending more time each week on childcare than women did in the 1960s, even while most are also working full-time.

THERE ARE NO GOOD OPTIONS

To be fair, emergencies are not the ideal time to sit down and calmly reallocate the division of labor in your relationships, especially not the mental load itself. And people socialized as men had their own burdens. They were likely to feel more pressure to keep providing economically and to be stoic about their emotions.

Pooja Lakshmin is a psychiatrist and author specializing in women's mental health, with a focus on how broken systems impact women's emotional lives. She told me the pandemic brought a huge increase in clinical depression and anxiety among her patients. Symptoms were more severe—anxious people were having panic attacks, and depressed people had thoughts of suicide. Lakshmin put this down to one big factor: the mental load and decision fatigue.

> It's a situation where there is no good option. There's no risk-free choice. When it comes to should I send my baby to daycare, is it OK for me to have a family member or hire a nanny if I can afford it, or should I be working at home full time and also trying to take care of an infant? There's been no real guide in terms of what is safe and what is not. So each family is having to really face the burden of these decisions. There's really no good answers and there's no 100 percent guarantee that you're making the right decision.

There Are No Good Options. TANGO. After I talked to Lakshmin, I wrote this acronym on the whiteboard on our refrigerator. It was to remind my husband and me, when we started to argue about outdoor dining or double masking or asking our house cleaner to come back, that neither of us was in fact the enemy. The pandemic was the enemy.

In Chapter 1, Rebecca Winthrop, the expert on "education in emergencies," said you can't hope for children to be resilient in a crisis unless you deeply support their caregivers. In 2020, women staggered under a teetering pile of extra work and responsibility, the conflict over who would actually do the work, the loss of social support, and the uncertainty, grief, and powerlessness of the situation. They reported a manifold increase in anxiety, loneliness, and depression. In one survey, nearly half of mothers with children home for remote learning reported their mental health had worsened, while just 30 percent of fathers said the same thing. (There may be a reporting bias in these numbers, as men are socialized not to talk about their mental health.)

Some women drank more. There was a sharp rise in alcoholic liver disease among younger women in their thirties. Some reported more drug use or weight gain. Mothers' reports of clinical insomnia, which correlated with reported anxiety about the pandemic, doubled in one Israeli survey.

Unavoidably, we took it out on our kids. In one study, caregiver depression rose and was the most significant predictor of self-reported lower-quality parenting. A lack of childcare and too much unstructured time also contributed. "They really described the loss of their typical support network and a lot of challenges around the breakdown of routines," says clinical psychologist Leslie Roos at the University of Manitoba, who has her own small children. "Relatives, other moms, going to the playground. All of that went away."

Maya, in San Francisco, experienced bouts of volatility, crying often. Dara, in New York, took Ambien in the early days to help her turn off her brain and sleep, harking back to her days as a medical resident. Heather, in St. Louis, smoked marijuana and turned to her positive affirmations.

Jeannie, in Oklahoma, had struggled with anxiety and depression for years. She went on and off different psychiatric medications during this time, put on weight, and experienced suicidal thoughts.

"It's easy to say I need help, but I don't know where to go," she told me. "School counselors tell me where to take my children, but for adults, it's not easily available. And I don't have time for that. So it's kind of like, I put myself on the back burner."

ELUSIVE SILVER LININGS

Some researchers, like Calarco, found women of higher socioeconomic status reported that the pandemic had a larger impact on their stress levels. This could be simply because women who were working-class had been through plenty of hard times before. It could also be because more privileged women started out with higher expectations of themselves both as workers and as mothers. "One of the things that really stuck out to us in the interviews was hearing the sense of failure that moms are experiencing. The moms were comparing themselves to these norms of ideal parenting and to these norms of the ideal worker." And they were falling short in both.

Not only were they comparing themselves to those norms, their bosses and other people in their lives were also doing it to them.

"One of our papers is called 'Let's Not Pretend It's Fun,'" says Calarco. "And that was from an interview with a mom who is working full-time from home during the pandemic. Her two-year-old daughter's childcare center closed. And her husband's also working full-time from home. And her mother-in-law kept sort of telling her, oh, you should be enjoying this time with your daughter, this is a special time. This is such a gift to have this extra time with your daughter."

Record scratch. It's a global pandemic! Not a vacation! "Hearing that from her mother-in-law and hearing that from other people in her life just gave her a sense of doubt and made her feel like a failure as a mother, and then also thinking about the work that she would normally be able to get done, feeling like a failure as a worker as well."

Some mothers were able to find that elusive silver lining. The key was that they weren't in the workforce. A team of researchers at the University of Chicago called up nearly six hundred low-income primary caregivers of toddlers in Chicago in May through July 2020. They asked: Do you feel more depressed or regularly overwhelmed? Are you yelling at your child a lot? Are you spending positive times, cuddling or playing a game just for fun?

Ariel Kalil and her coauthors expected to find worse mental health and impaired family functioning. In most cases, as in Roos's study, this was true. Stress was up and depression symptoms were more common. Under stress, parents yelled, they got impatient, they withdrew from their children.

But 9 percent of Kalil's sample was different. They reported experiencing a job loss with no income loss. Federal CARES Act money or some other circumstance created something approaching paid parental leave.

These mothers reported fewer adverse impacts on their mental health and more positive interactions with their children: more cuddles, more games. "Even during this pandemic, where you have this big kind of shock of an unexpected increase in time" spent caregiving, Kalil said, "parents really seem to find the value in this. There are rewards."

Patricia identifies strongly as a working woman, and she never left her job. But she did find some rewards in spending more time at home. "I feel like I've gotten a lot of lost time that was stolen from me," she said. She hadn't had much maternity leave with either of her two boys. "I had my first child July 27; I went right back to work August 25." She said she was mindful of stereotypes about Black women and didn't want to go on unemployment, which was the only way she could have afforded to stay home. "So it's been invaluable that, you know, the world stopped and paused, because it gave me a moment to do so much since March. I spent more time with my kids, with my husband. We've really worked on our marriage, talking to each other and just hanging out."

Patricia had her ups and downs, but she rededicated herself to self-care. She found a therapist. She had been gaining weight, so she started working with a personal trainer, too, someone she met in the neighborhood. "I want to come out of quarantine as a sexy butterfly," she told me.

CUSTODY DISPUTES

COVID created "emotionally devastating" circumstances for co-parents living in separate houses, in the words of one family lawyer. Ex-partners butted heads over visitation agreements because they were worried about the risk of travel, because one parent was an essential worker or lived in a COVID hotspot, because of a particularly vulnerable household member, or simply because of the added risk of moving between two different households. They argued over different rules and risk tolerances—over masking, indoor playdates, sending kids to school and daycare. Family courts were working less efficiently during the pandemic, making it harder to get clarity on disputes. If visitation stopped or decreased, the parent with primary custody, usually the mom, was left with even more responsibility than before.

THE PILEUP

The case is pretty clear: Most mothers during COVID did more domestic labor than fathers did. They did more household chores, more caregiving, more homeschooling, more decision making, while mostly continuing to work for wages as well. They tended to worry about COVID more. And it all took a heavy toll on them, economically, mentally, and physically—and on their children. And they blamed themselves for all of it.

As I sat in my own sometimes chaotic house, trading off meetings with my own husband and wondering what to cook for dinner, I read story after story after story about the disproportionate burden falling on mothers. I was silently screaming.

A pure rational-actor theory of economics would predict that a two-earner family, at a time of massive economic uncertainty, would adjust the division of paid and unpaid labor to keep both earners in the workforce whenever possible. Forcing mothers out of the workforce, or even forcing them to downshift, can be economically ruinous for individual households and for society as a whole. Yes, men usually earn more than their female partners. But most two-parent households in the United States still rely on both parents' incomes to get by. And leaving the workforce, even temporarily, causes a shock not only to immediate household income but to retirement savings and future progress in the workforce.

On the emotional side of the ledger, you might also predict that husbands would go above and beyond to prevent their partners from becoming disproportionately insomniac, drunken, depressed, and anxious. Or at least you'd expect that fathers would do what was necessary so that their genetic offspring weren't being yelled at and potentially treated harshly by moms at the end of their rope.

Employers could and should have done more. Governments, particularly the US government, could and should have done more. But what I keep coming back to is the call that never ever came from inside the house. Heterosexual couples overwhelmingly tacitly agreed to sacrifice mothers' earnings and their sanity to the pandemic. It was a decision as shortsighted as pulling down the timbers of your own house to burn for fuel in a snowstorm.

It's funny, but amid the dozens and dozens of surveys and media articles about women being "forced" from the workforce—like it was an act of nature!—I didn't find the same level of curiosity about why more dads didn't step up. I didn't find lots of polls or interview-based studies where they asked men, "How are you OK with your wife working herself to shreds and worrying herself to pieces while you sit on your Zoom calls with your noise-canceling headphones? How do YOU sleep at night?"

FRED AND WILMA FLINTSTONE IS A MYTH

I'm going to go back to history to try to answer that question. Actually, to prehistory.

The concept of a single-breadwinner nuclear family is pretty novel. For tens of thousands of years, in hunter-gatherer and then agrarian societies, the household was the place of production as well as reproduction. Men, women, and children lived in multigenerational groups. They all did many useful things, including caregiving, according to their abilities, age, and other factors.

I think most of us grew up believing that cavewoman Wilma Flintstone foraged for berries while her caveman hubby, Fred, clubbed the saber-toothed tigers. Lately, that simplistic scenario has been challenged. A paper published in late 2020 documented a nine-thousand-year-old burial site in South America that included women hunters. Similar sites have been found throughout the Americas, in a proportion suggesting that strong young women and strong young men actually hunted big game together in roughly equal numbers, at least in that part of the world.

Whatever the case, it wasn't until industrialization in the late nineteenth and early twentieth centuries that most families were made to depend on cash wages outside the home. These were earned over long hours by young unmarried women, children, and men. Meanwhile, it became more typical for women with children to stay home with the other household tasks. This cleaving of life into two separate spheres was accompanied by a whole lot of Victorian ideology about how "natural" it was, which is your tip-off that it was completely manufactured and brand new.

The problem was, not every household with children happened to have a wage-earning man.

PAY MOTHERS OR TAKE CHILDREN?

One response to this reality, as covered in Chapter 3, was the nineteenth-century day nursery movement. But even many of the philanthropic women who built these charity nurseries thought it was a shame that a mother should have to leave her children to work.

Self-proclaimed philanthropists often favored helping children by themselves: putting them in orphanages, placing "foundlings" with richer families, or shipping them off on an Orphan Train. The elitist fantasy here is that you are improving society as a whole by rescuing children from their inferior families.

In the first decade of the twentieth century, a new idea took hold: publicly subsidizing mothers to stay home with their own children. As the delegates of the first White House Conference on Care of Dependent Children in 1909 put it, "Home life is the finest and highest product of civilization.... Children should not be deprived of it except for urgent and compelling reasons." And therefore, "children of reasonably efficient and deserving mothers who are without the support of the normal breadwinners should, as a rule, be kept with their parents."

Two key words are doing a lot of work here: "normal" and "deserving." The ideology of American welfare from the beginning is that people have to deserve it. And it can't be so generous that it upsets what's "normal" according to patriarchy: men as breadwinners. And these deserving mothers were overwhelmingly seen as white.

Still, the idea was compelling, even revolutionary. As sociologist Theda Skocpol argues in her 1992 book *Protecting Soldiers and Mothers*, the pension metaphor was crucial in establishing who was deserving of government largesse. Up until this point in American history, only veterans of war had successfully laid a mass claim on public funds for their support. So mothers were compared to those veterans. She quotes President Teddy Roosevelt in 1912: "A pension given to such a mother...who has had to be both father and mother, is as much a matter of right as any pension given to the most deserving soldier."

However, the comparatively lean federal government didn't step in to fund these pensions. It was two male judges in the emerging legal area of juvenile court, E. E. Porterfield in Kansas City, Missouri, and Merritt Pinckney in Cook County, Illinois, who successfully lobbied state legislatures to create the first two mothers' pension laws. Eventually, by 1934, a year after the New Deal began, there were "mother's aid" laws in forty-six states, the District of Columbia, plus the territories of Alaska and Hawaii.

The first government-sponsored welfare program in the United States, mothers' pensions were a historical fork in the road.

The mothers' pension, more than a hundred years ago, actually put a dollar value on women's care work. Wages for housework! This was considered a radical idea at the fringes of feminism in the 1970s, and fifty years later it remains radical and fringe.

The public discourse framed care work as noble, even a public service. "If she has given a citizen to the nation, the nation owes something to her," proclaimed a Mrs. G. Harris Robertson at the 1911 Second International Congress on Child Welfare.

And the program made a big difference in the lives of children. A 2014 paper found "male children of accepted applicants lived one year longer than those of rejected mothers. They also obtained one-third more years of schooling, were less likely to be underweight, and had higher income in adulthood than children of rejected mothers."

Imagine if we'd continued on this path of recognizing and adequately funding care work. Imagine the dignity and the pride. Imagine what our country might have looked like after several generations of children grew up without knowing the bite of poverty and parental desperation. Imagine the wholeness of body, mind, and spirit those children could have passed on to their children, their children's children, and to us.

But now we have to crash back to earth. Mothers' pensions were usually funded locally, at the county or city level. There were concerns about "encouraging divorce" and removing the impetus to work for wages, so these pensions were never set at an amount a mother and child could actually live on. And, during the New Deal, FDR used the existence of these pensions as an excuse not to give more money to his newly created Aid to Dependent Children program.

As happened with the school lunch program around the same time, in the middle of the twentieth century, local authorities administered mothers' aid programs with a heavy dose of racial discrimination and moral judgment, attitudes that also served the purpose of keeping spending down. At least eight states, mostly in the South, had rules regulating access to welfare based on mothers' personal lives. Welfare workers made home visits to see whether mothers had a man in the house.

In what became known as the "Louisiana Incident," in 1960, the state expelled twenty-three thousand children from its welfare rolls all at once, for the crime of being born out of wedlock. Most were Black. Laura Briggs, in her book *Taking Children*, argues that this move was in part retaliation against integrationists. If the civil rights movement was going to put little children like Ruby Bridges in the middle of the fight for equality, well, the Dixiecrats could spotlight Black children, too, by taking away their means of survival. The move backfired on the segregationists from a PR perspective, Briggs argues. Moderate groups like the Urban League created Operation Save the Babies, a mutual aid effort to feed and clothe these suddenly destitute children.

The Louisiana Incident caused such a commotion that the federal secretary of the Department of Health, Education, and Welfare, Arthur Flemming, felt called upon to put in place what became known as the "Flemming rule." In sum, it said, if you don't want to help a poor family because you don't judge the mother to be "deserving," that's fine with us. But you can't just leave them alone. The rule led to an explosion of child removals in the Black community, which Briggs has called "the browning of child welfare." It laid the groundwork for the situation we see today, where one in four of the children placed in foster care is there for neglect, which typically means simply poverty. Things like coming to school without a coat in winter or with nothing but a bag of chips for lunch or missing a dentist appointment or two because of unreliable transportation can trigger a call from a school or a doctor's office to child welfare and from there to a home being declared inadequate.

A version of this same policing and shaming of mothers persists today under the 1996 welfare reform act. States are required to collect information on children's biological fathers in order to pursue those men for child support—child support the states then pocket as reimbursement for welfare assistance. So applying for much-needed help requires women to talk about their sex lives and disclose personal information that can lead to the impoverishment or prosecution of their children's fathers. ProPublica reported that during the pandemic, federal and state governments intercepted an estimated $684 million in coronavirus stimulus money and other funds intended for low-income fathers.

WELFARE RIGHTS AND THE QUIET REVOLUTION

Around the same time as the Louisiana Incident, a labor organizer and community activist who was the daughter of a sharecropper fell ill. Johnnie Tillmon reluctantly signed up for public assistance to support her six children. She ended up cofounding and chairing the National Welfare Rights Organization. In 1972, in the pages of the newly founded *Ms.* magazine, she laid it out for her fellow women's libbers in an essay whose lede still socks you in the gut. "I'm a woman. I'm a black woman. I'm a poor woman. I'm a fat woman. I'm a middle-aged woman. And I'm on welfare. In this country, if you're any one of those things you count less as a human being. If you're all those things, you don't count at all. Except as a statistic."

"For a lot of middle-class women in this country, Women's Liberation is a matter of concern. For women on welfare it's a matter of survival," Tillmon explained, outlining the indignities of welfare: "Welfare is like a super-sexist marriage. You trade in a man for *the* man. But you can't divorce him if he treats you bad. He can divorce you, of course, cut you off anytime he wants. But in that case, *he* keeps the kids, not you. *The* man runs everything."

The mothers of NWRO wanted "*the* man" off their backs. They didn't want intrusion in their personal lives. They didn't want their children taken away on the slimmest pretext. They wanted "guaranteed adequate income," for everyone, without scrutiny, control, or judgment. Something more like Social Security. Or like a veteran's pension.

Another fork in the road. This was an era of sweeping social changes and major new federal programs. We'd just begun an entire war on poverty. The women's movement and the civil rights movement could have united behind a simplified program that actually eradicated poverty among children, the way expanded Social Security and the new Medicare program were beginning to do for the elderly.

But in the 1970s, something else was on the rise. What the feminist economist Claudia Goldin called in a famous 2006 paper of the same title: "The Quiet Revolution."

Kathryn Anne Edwards, an economist at the RAND Corporation, is the one who filled me in on this, so I'm going to let her take over for a bit: "Her thesis of a quiet revolution is that with very little outward change to policy, women completely revolutionized the way that they approached [paid] work. And they did so on three levels, in how they viewed career as part of their identity, in the time horizons for making decisions about their job, and how they saw their earnings fitting into the household."

Identity: Is your job part of your self-discovery? One of the determinants of life satisfaction? Or just a paycheck? In physician Dara Kass's words, "I am making a very, very meaningful difference in people's lives at a time when they are scared. And that's a gift....I've had a purpose."

Horizon: Meaning, when you're getting your education, do you see yourself working full-time for many years, or just for a few years and part-time? You invest accordingly.

Earnings fitting into the household: Are you the de facto second income, an equal partner, or the breadwinner whose career takes precedence?

"Thinking about the '50s," says Edwards. "Women would work, but they would often quit when they got married or when they had kids. And it was very much a secondary decision—secondary to their husbands' earnings. And it wasn't supposed to be for their whole life. It was just something they did for a while. So [Goldin] brings together evidence to talk about how career becomes part of women's identity. And it coincides with, you know, almost thirty years of undeterred increase in women's labor force participation."

For three decades, in other words, beginning in the 1970s, women tried to pull ourselves up by our bootstraps, no matter how impossible that might be. We did everything we could to demonstrate dedication to our careers. We caught up to and surpassed men in higher education. We delayed our marriages and had fewer children with the help of legalized birth control and abortion. We started working young and we kept at it for decades.

THE QUIET REVOLUTION AND THE FEMINIST AGENDA

Hearing this from Edwards was a lightning flash for me. I suddenly realized how the pursuit of the quiet revolution in the workplace dictated the feminist agenda for half a century.

The marquee feminist issues that I've been aware of since I was a little girl are equal pay, equal representation in leadership at the C-suite level and in the halls of government, reproductive rights, beauty standards, sexual harassment, and sexual violence. All worthy causes. This is the agenda of the quiet revolutionaries—upwardly mobile, primarily white and straight women who are conscious of themselves as targets of sexual objectification and for whom the ultimate goal was the corner office. Pantsuit Nation.

Childcare, the removal of children by the state, guaranteed adequate income, or at least some less racist, less sexist, less intrusive, more adequate form of welfare—none of these have been close to the center of the kind of feminism that gets the most media attention.

We saw this disconnect in 1996, when President Bill Clinton executed his pledge to "end welfare as we know it." At the time, 95 percent of welfare recipients were women. Gender and poverty scholar Gwendolyn Mink argued in 1998: "The Personal Responsibility Act is the most aggressive invasion of women's rights in this century, and most women did little to resist it. Many feminists actually endorsed the new law's core principles—mainly, that poor single mothers should move from welfare to work and into financial relationships with their children's fathers."

What happened instead with welfare reform was a drop in the number of families receiving cash aid, a rise in child poverty and homelessness, and a growth in the numbers of the working poor.

As journalist Lauren Sandler describes in her 2020 book *This Is All I Got*, which follows a single mother's quest for survival in and out of shelters and affordable housing in New York City, welfare reform often means in practice that you drop off your child at the home of another woman living at the edge of poverty, just so you can sit all day in a job center waiting for work that never comes.

Or as Katherine Boo, writing for the *New Yorker* two decades earlier, in 2001, famously put it, "It is possible to see welfare reform as a Ponzi scheme whose currency is children."

ARE YOU "*THE* MAN"?

The lack of solidarity can be uncomfortably personal. Mothers who gain economic power increasingly outsource our household labor.

Higher pay means you can order takeout and hire cleaners and babysitters. Most of the time this means hiring other women, especially women of color and immigrants, who earn less than you do. You might be a staunch feminist when you're asking for a promotion. But after hours, are you *"the* man," haggling with your nanny and paying her cash under the table, no overtime?

THE QUIET REVOLUTION HITS AN INVISIBLE LIMIT

"We've hit some kind of limit to how much women participate in the labor force, just based on their own willpower, " Kathryn Anne Edwards said. "There are serious barriers to having two parents participate fully in the labor market."

We could go no further without social support of the type that is common across wealthy countries: guaranteed paid leave, subsidized childcare. Even Japan, one of the most traditionalist and patriarchal affluent societies in the world, passed us in 2017, with the assist of a falling birthrate.

By the way, Edwards took my call from inside a closet. She and her husband couldn't afford full-time childcare, so they were getting by with a part-time sitter.

"I am not the aloof observer of this year's consequences," she told me. "I'm an active participant in everything I said is going on with women. I was on maternity leave when the pandemic hit and I rolled straight from maternity into a pandemic."

The pink-pussy-hat, grrl-power feminism I was raised on doesn't speak to this moment. We have a stalled revolution on our hands. Women haven't made gains in the workforce for two decades. We still haven't ascended to the presidency in the United States or held more than one in four Senate seats.

And we can't do it without solidarity, public programs, *and* men stepping up.

THE END OF LEAN IN?

I talked to Marianne Cooper about this. She is a sociologist and the lead researcher of *Lean In: Women, Work, and the Will to Lead*.

That was the blockbuster, enormously influential 2013 book by Facebook executive Sheryl Sandberg, one of the highest-ranking women in Silicon Valley. It urged women to rededicate themselves to the quiet revolution.

Success, as the subtitle had it, was a matter not of systemic change but of personal "will." Implicitly, by this model, the women's movement succeeds when we control 250 of the Fortune 500 companies. This is a vision of feminism that asks virtually nothing of the government. It whites out structural inequalities. It has little to say to women like the nannies who accompanied Sandberg on private jets, making her own work-life balance possible.

Cooper and I happened to talk on the day of the Capitol insurrection, January 6, 2021. A man named Richard Barnett was putting his feet up on House Speaker Nancy Pelosi's desk, showing dangerous contempt for one of the most powerful women in government. This, after voters picked one of the oldest men ever to run for president over an entire field of highly qualified women in the primary, with some polling suggesting that voters believed *other* voters would never accept a woman in the top spot.

Cooper told me we were in a New Deal moment. It was time for collective solutions.

> The resources and ways of managing that a lot of women had kind of cobbled together…evaporated literally overnight. And it just revealed such shortcomings in how we're all trying to figure this out on our own, and that that's not the best system.
>
> And so, despite vast inequalities among women themselves, I think that the similarity of that experience could actually cause people to see policy in a different way. We need public policy solutions. We need a government that works for everybody.

So I think there's a possibility now. I know the power of neoliber-
alism and the power of meritocracy and the power of individualism,
its ideologies, to really prevent that from happening.

But if there was ever a time for some real change, some real policy
changes, it would be now.

Stirring words! I was surprised and seized my opening. "As someone who's been so identified with *Lean In*, I mean, is that not an
example of meritocracy and individualism?" I asked.

Cooper responded, "[Sandberg] certainly isn't the first person to
have written a book about how to individually try to figure out your
ways through unequal systems."

I told her I didn't want to set up a "straw-woman" argument, but
this was personal for me. "As someone who graduated college in
2002, I feel like the image of what ambitious women in my generation were supposed to do had a lot to do with succeeding by working
harder, proving myself, and not internalizing stereotypes. And if I
made enough money, I could pay for work-life balance." The quiet
revolution roadmap.

"I've given talks on discrimination and bias and how basically
most women are kind of fucked and women walk away from that
horribly depressed," countered Cooper. "I'm not sure it's the most
helpful thing in the world to say that if you're marrying a man, the
odds that your relationship is going to be equal, especially once you
have children, is like slim to none. I don't know of a couple that bal-
ances things equally. And I'm in feminist scholarship circles. So the
point is that people want to know how to navigate these systems and
they don't want the answer to be, you have to wait until we pass all
these laws and we enforce these laws and all of these things until you
can actually get your shot at whatever it is that you want to get your
shot at. And so therefore, people need survival strategies right now."

Until there's a global catastrophe, followed by an insurrection, and
your survival strategies evaporate overnight, I guess. Then maybe, just
maybe, it is the time to call for big structural change.

When I think about the kind of political work the moment calls for, I'm haunted by something C. Nicole Mason at the Institute for Women's Policy Research (IWPR) told me. She happens to be one of the few Black women in charge of a major think tank in Washington. "I actually think this has been quite a unifying moment because women have realized that, like, the system wasn't working for us at all. You know, corporate women to grocery store clerks, they've all sort of said, you know, like, I thought it was just me. The pandemic has sort of said, wait a minute, it's not you. It's actually a system that may not be working for women."

But, she said, IWPR surveyed women to ask whether they agreed that the pandemic was a unifying moment. Do women need each other now more than ever?

"Forty percent said yes, but I can tell you that Black and Latina women said yes by 60 percent or 50 percent, and white women were like 30 percent. They voted for Trump so it doesn't shock me."

DAD SOS

The other part that I'm still stewing over is the part where 97 percent of the married heterosexual cisgender dads are MIA in this. Biden, or any president, can't fix that.

The unequal division of domestic labor during the pandemic, as women were driven from the workforce, occurred even in countries that had a decent safety net for caregivers. In Australia, nearly a tenth of women exited the workforce. In the UK, mothers with small children were 10 percentage points more likely than fathers to lose their jobs. In Japan, women lost jobs at nearly twice the rate of men. In Germany, one-third of families relied exclusively on mothers as caregivers when other options were closed, whereas just 4 to 6 percent relied on fathers. But the government's generous furlough program kept women from losing their jobs at higher rates than men.

I reflect on how the #MeToo movement asked women to confront the men in their lives. It got personal; it got uncomfortable.

There were real consequences in relationships, not just in the public sphere.

The Black Lives Matter uprising of 2020 also was framed in part as a personal racial reckoning on a broader scale than ever seen before. Many white people and non-Black people of color thought about the role that anti-Blackness played in their own lives and relationships. They bought tens of thousands of books and initiated conversations in schools, communities, workplaces. That phenomenon had its cringey side (like white men who Venmoed their Black ex-girlfriends out of the blue, as reported by the podcast *Reply All* in June 2020).

Movement activists were asking for structural changes, not just changes of heart. But I respect the impulse, at least, to square the political with the personal.

Mothers, and all primary caregivers, need to pursue personal reckonings along with political change. For one thing, when we're doing too much at home, it leaves us with no time to fight for political change.

HOW TO NEGOTIATE A BETTER DEAL AT HOME

Linda Hirshman, in her 2006 manifesto *Get to Work*, advises career-minded women to marry either a downwardly mobile, less educated, perhaps younger man or an older, semiretired one. That's one strategy, and I have to say I've seen it work.

Brigid Schulte, a journalist for the *Washington Post*, published a book in 2014 called *Overwhelmed: Work, Love, and Play When No One Has the Time* and revealed that, actually, it was moms who didn't have the time, because dads were taking it. She started the Better Life Lab at the liberal think tank New America to try to engage families in negotiating better divisions of labor: through chore charts, shared calendars, and family meetings.

Unfortunately, it often falls to mothers to do the emotional labor of introducing, selling, and enforcing these systems, an imbalance Schulte, when I talked to her, didn't have a good solution for.

Eve Rodsky was working as a mediator, had a toddler and a newborn, and was living a privileged but hectic life in Los Angeles. One day she was driving to a client meeting with her breast pump and diaper bag when her husband texted her, "I'm surprised you didn't get blueberries."

Lesser mortals might get divorced. Rodsky crowdsourced a spreadsheet with contributions from hundreds of women about their divisions of domestic labor and wrote a best-selling 2019 book called *Fair Play*, which she also turned into a card game that helps each partner visualize the work they are doing to keep the household running. Her mission is to make mothers' invisible labor visible and to get women to stop being "complicit in their own oppression."

During the pandemic Rodsky formed an initiative called Careforce, made up of policymakers, business leaders, academics, and other opinionated types. They're trying to move the conversation more toward collective solutions, while not overlooking the role of the personal.

In the end, work is required on many different levels. To benefit children, we need a solution for mothers, fathers, and all caregivers, paid and unpaid. We need public initiatives and we need personal reimagining. We need to see the unseen work.

"We don't give a shit about mothers. Right? We erase them," Rodsky told me. It made me think again of those Victorian mothers with the black cloths over their heads, a dark joke on the erasure of caregiving. Hidden mother photography is a real-life illustration of famous remarks by Donald Winnicott, one of the foremost theorists of attachment. "There is no such thing as a baby," he writes. "A baby alone doesn't exist." What exists, in his view, is a "nursing couple": a baby plus, as his phrase implies, a mother.

And actually limiting it only to that dyad, or even the nuclear family, is another kind of erasure, another kind of hiding. Babies don't grow up by themselves. Mothers and "nursing couples" don't thrive without partners, kin, friends, and public structures of care.

8   SCHOOLS

But whether it's Dr. Fauci or anybody else, a lot of people got it wrong. They talked about don't wear masks, and now they say wear masks. Although some people say don't wear masks.... Now there is, by the way, a lot of people who don't want to wear masks. There are a lot of people who think that masks are not good.

> —Trump in an ABC News town hall, September 15, 2020

September 22, 2020, US death toll reaches 200,000

April and June, Jeannie's twins, were sent home with a COVID exposure on the very first day of in-person third grade in the fall of 2020. Pretty soon, she, and they, were all feeling sick.

"I thought I prepared them. I told them, no matter what, leave your mask on all day," she told me over Zoom from her white-slipcovered sectional sofa, where she was quarantining, feverish. "I thought, they need to set an example. Wear a mask, maybe everybody else will too. It didn't happen."

In fact, some children came in wearing hand-crocheted, open-work lace masks—a crafty-grandma middle finger to the CDC. This was Oklahoma, one of the reddest states in the country. President Trump had chosen Tulsa, in June, for his first in-person campaign event since March 2020. Several high-profile Republican attendees got COVID after the largely unmasked indoors event. One, politician Herman Cain, died. And the number of daily COVID-19 cases in the state tripled in the thirty days following the rally.

"I feel like at some point in the summer, Oklahomans just decided we were finished with the pandemic and that we were just going to live normally," Jeannie told me. "We've been just going full throttle ever since. A lot of people just say they still don't believe it's dangerous or real. Getting those people to just do the right thing, it's not going to happen."

Jeannie and the twins all tested negative. But Jeannie spent all ten days of quarantine home on the couch, struggling to support her remote students. For several weeks, she had brain fog, coughed, and smelled a strange chemical smell.

Despite everything, Jeannie and her family had found some bright spots at home during the summer of 2020. Although Jeannie had pretty much given up on virtual schooling in the spring, she regained the energy to give the girls their regular summer enrichment lessons in the tidy dining room. The walls were lined with bookshelves full of workbooks, and with Jeannie's many photographs of the children posed in fanciful costumes—as sunflowers, Einstein, or in Day of the Dead makeup. She took some of the family grant money sent by the Cherokee Nation and set up a playhouse in the backyard with the girls. They decorated it in a mid-century modern style, with a cat motif. They also got a new trampoline.

Things were tenser with the boys, her teens. When they were home, they were in their rooms. For Rob, thirteen, that was pretty much always. He was chatting while playing Xbox with his friends, except when they were hanging out, indoors, in person, without him. "I'm not really involved in a lot of stuff with my friends. Like, they get to hang out a lot because their parents don't care as much about COVID, I guess."

Julian, sixteen, was working nearly full-time at Sonic. He'd been promoted to assistant manager, getting a raise to eight dollars an hour. He had a girlfriend too.

For the fall, Jeannie made a complicated plan. To limit the family's total exposure, Julian and Rob would stay remote. The girls would go to school in person, because Jeannie judged that it was too much to leave ten-year-old Ruby in charge of the "babies" all day.

"I felt like I had to sacrifice someone. They got put into the public school, into the classroom."

While she was making these stressful decisions, work was equally stressful. In the spring the school had fallen back on "emergency remote learning." Jeannie's district used paper packets because so many students weren't connected, and relaxed grading and other requirements to the point where they were nearly nonexistent.

The fall was a different story. To their credit, with the help of federal funding, the district had gotten mobile hotspots and laptops out to almost every student. This was a big effort around the country, and it made a lot of progress; a survey in the spring of 2021 suggested that more than nine out of ten families with school-aged children now had at least one computer at home, with the biggest increase coming among families at the poverty line.

The hotspots didn't always work well for her students who lived out on rural roads with little cell phone signal. But for fall 2020, Jeannie's school still expected teachers to create full-fledged virtual lessons, including recorded videos. And they were also expected to teach their regular classes in person, without so much as an extra planning period during the day to grade the work of remote students or answer their constant questions. "I've been really frustrated about that and almost belligerent," an ill Jeannie told me. "It's just chaos. I feel like it's failed."

MOST US STUDENTS STAYED REMOTE IN FALL 2020

Failure and chaos, frustration and belligerence were common among educators, parents, and kids in the fall of 2020.

The federal CARES Act passed at the end of March 2020 earmarked $13.5 billion for schools. That sounds like a lot of money until you realize that public schools spend more than $600 billion annually.

Despite frequent public statements from President Trump on the importance of opening schools ("OPEN THE SCHOOLS!!!" he tweeted on August 4), Congress didn't appropriate any additional money to help them do it. The next, much larger, installment of coronavirus aid money to schools didn't come until December, far too late to plan for opening in the fall. And the money took even longer to actually get to classrooms.

This meant in the fall of 2020, public schools didn't have a lot of extra money lying around to set up outdoor learning spaces, conduct frequent rapid testing, or hire staff to reduce class sizes, all steps that might have made it safer to come back.

We don't have comprehensive national data on school reopening plans during this time. That's because the federal Department of Education under Secretary Betsy DeVos specifically declined to collect it.

A mom-and-pop data company called Burbio, based in New Jersey, stepped into the breach. Dennis Roche, his wife Julie, and a small team published a regular "school reopening tracker" that scraped a large sample of district websites from every county in the United States.

The school year started slow, with last-minute delays and changes of plan. By mid-October 2020, Burbio found 42 percent of students were attending schools that offered only remote learning. A further 34.7 percent were enrolled in schools with in-person learning five days a week, like Jeannie's. The remainder went to schools that offered in-person learning part-time, staggering groups of students to comply with the CDC's six-foot distancing rule.

Remote learning was the rule in California, Washington State, and in big-city, blue-state school districts across the country. Full-time in-person learning was more common in the Sun Belt, in states like Texas, Georgia, and Florida.

Even the schools that were teaching in person were almost always offering a virtual option at the same time. So coast to coast, remote students most likely outnumbered in-person students throughout the fall.

The rest of the year was a roller coaster. Districts opened up gradually in person throughout the fall. As the terrifying, worse-than-ever second wave of the pandemic crested, they went remote again, generally for several weeks. Thanksgiving break blurred into Christmas and New Year's and January.

By the spring, some districts that had not yet opened in person started to tentatively try. But they found the longer they had waited, the fewer families came back to the classroom. When the Biden administration finally released national figures, they found 68 percent of Asian American, 58 percent of Black, and 56 percent of Hispanic fourth graders were still learning entirely remotely in February 2021. Conversely, nearly half of white fourth graders were learning in person—full-time, not even hybrid. In all, close to half of US students were out of physical school for almost a full calendar year. These children were disproportionately children of color, urban, and low income.

This back-to-school chapter picks apart how the United States failed to get so many students back in classrooms for so long and what happened to those who went back and those who stayed home.

HEALTH AUTHORITIES RECOMMENDED OPENING SCHOOLS IN THE FALL

In the spring of 2020, schools were closed out of caution. It was relatively uncontroversial. It happened almost everywhere in the world— although European countries started opening up within several weeks, and Sweden's never closed.

The 2020–2021 school year, the subject of this chapter, was a whole different animal. Our peer countries committed to opening schools whenever possible. Politics held sway over science in the United States' weak, decentralized, inequitably funded school system.

THE DIRECT IMPACT OF THE VIRUS ON CHILDREN

Through the end of the summer of 2020, the United States had suffered an appalling two hundred thousand COVID deaths. By any measure we were doing a terrible job controlling the pandemic. And fewer than two hundred of those victims were under the age of twenty-one. So it was clear the risk to children from the disease directly remained low even in the context of barely controlled spread.

Six-year-old Gigi Morse died of the disease in August 2020 in Jackson, Tennessee. According to the *Washington Post*, "She was a dynamo of a kid who loved Froot Loops and was obsessed with all things 'Frozen'—the songs, the characters." Gigi was adopted from Ukraine at the age of three. She had epilepsy, autism, and hydrocephaly. A UK study found that about half of child COVID-19 deaths occurred in those, like Gigi, with complex health-care needs.

Her six-year-old brother was the one who discovered her body. "The virus didn't kill anyone else in the Morse family, but Gigi's mother says it might as well have. The pain does not ebb. The guilt gnaws at them constantly," wrote the *Post* reporter.

The loss of each child is overwhelming, and no words can measure it accurately.

It's also true that the scientific consensus had solidified by the fall of 2020: COVID was dramatically less dangerous for children than for adults. Furthermore, evidence mounted that putting kids in classrooms, with the right precautions, did not have to mean increasing cases in their households or the broader community. That basic dynamic did not change with the subsequent variants.

Another complication in thinking about the risks of COVID infections to the young was "long COVID." In adults this vexing syndrome seemed to present similarly to other autoimmune disorders and ailments like chronic fatigue syndrome. Some children and especially teenagers reported serious and debilitating symptoms like intense fatigue, brain fog, and lingering breathing problems for more than six months after infection.

The burning question was exactly how many. There were major limitations in the research into 2022. Some studies found almost no difference in reported symptoms whether people had actually tested positive for COVID or not. And there were researchers who pointed out that lingering symptoms like a cough are common to many viral illnesses like flu. The potential psychosocial dimensions of long COVID remained a matter of huge controversy. Long-haulers organized, participated in patient advocacy, and pushed for research and treatments, and so did the parents of children who were identified as long-haulers. Specialized clinics popped up to treat them. One, at Yale University, reported in November 2021 that the majority of its patients recovered within a few months.

IT WAS "INSANE" TO CLOSE SCHOOLS, ONE DOCTOR SAYS

"I think it's safe" was Dara Kass's judgment of schooling as of the fall of 2020, reflecting a growing medical consensus. "You need to look at community spread. You need to look at your policies in schools— mask wearing is critically important. And you need to make sure that your kids understand the world we're living in right now. But in an intentional environment like a school, with mask wearing and the right protocols in place, we're not seeing transmission among kids."

For her own family, it's fair to note, Dara was more cautious. She kept her older two children learning remotely in the fall, to limit the family's overall exposure. She created a full-time eight-person "pandemic pod" in her basement for her younger son, Sammy, her "transplant kid," trusting she'd be able to control his environment better that way.

"It was so insane for people to close schools," Danny Benjamin tells me. He's one of the top research pediatricians in the country, chair of the National Institute of Child Health and Human Development's Pediatric Trials Network, and cochair of the ABC Science Collaborative. Funded by the National Institutes of Health, the collaborative worked with districts all over the country to provide evidence-based support for decision making around COVID mitigation.

"We had all this preliminary data from health care" that universal mask wearing limited transmission of this virus, he says. "It's respiratory physiology. Why would the virus act differently in school than it does in hospitals?"

Unfortunately, this interview took place with the benefit of hindsight, in October 2021.

THE RISKS OF KEEPING CHILDREN HOME

Reopening schools was never just about the risks to children or their families of getting sick from COVID. It was about the risks to children of staying home. As 2020 wore on, experts on children's well-being around the globe, such as UNICEF, the World Health Organization (WHO), the American Academy of Pediatrics, and the Organisation for Economic Co-operation and Development, got louder. They all warned that the danger to children of prolonged school closures was outweighing the danger of opening them.

"COVID-19 appears to have a limited direct burden on children's health, accounting for about 8.5% of reported cases globally, and very few deaths," reported the WHO in September 2020. "In contrast, school closures have clear negative impacts on child health, education and development, family income and the overall economy."

"The evidence available strongly suggests that transmission resulting in symptomatic infection of either children or adults is uncommon in schools" was the statement of the European Union's equivalent of the CDC in August 2020. However, it cited "various negative impacts on children's wellbeing, learning opportunities and safety caused by school closures."

By December it got even more direct: "There is a general consensus that the decision to close schools to control the COVID-19 pandemic should be used as a last resort. The negative physical, mental health and educational impact of proactive school closures on children, as well as the economic impact on society more broadly, would likely outweigh the benefits."

Many countries across Europe and Asia committed to opening schools for the fall. On one end of the spectrum, Iceland and Sweden never closed primary schools, and Switzerland reopened its schools after just forty-one days.

During subsequent waves, European countries sometimes closed again, but they kept prioritizing schools for opening. For example, during a surge in cases in the fall of 2020, Germany shut down restaurants, bars, theaters, gyms, tattoo parlors, and legal brothels, while keeping schools open. In mid-December through January, France imposed restrictions including a nationwide curfew but kept schools and nurseries open.

The upshot was that students in peer countries of the United States, including the UK, Israel, France, Germany, Italy, Spain, New Zealand, across Scandinavia, most parts of Australia, Japan, South Korea, Thailand, Vietnam, and China, ended up with far more weeks of full-time in-person learning by the end of the school year than most students here.

The US racked up fifteen months shut to millions of students, putting it in a league with Brazil, Chile, and India. All the way into the spring of 2021, in cities like Boston, San Francisco, and New York, schools were closed or offering only limited in-person hours to a fraction of students while indoor dining, bars, gyms, and other businesses were all open.

The question of this chapter is why.

The first-order explanation is clearly that this country did an exceptionally terrible job managing the pandemic. If we'd prevented transmission, we could've saved a universe of lives and reopened our schools after nine weeks like New Zealand did.

However, the subject of this book is not epidemic control but how the United States failed children.

Dimitri Christakis is the editor in chief of the pediatrics journal of the American Medical Association.

He saw evidence COVID was not very dangerous to children but the lack of in-person schooling was. And he became a passionate advocate for reopening schools wherever possible. In the fall of 2020, he told me:

> We failed children in three important ways. You know, first and foremost, that we have done such a terrible job containing this pandemic.
>
> Secondly, that we closed schools summarily and abruptly without any good plan about how to transition to distance learning and without adequate infrastructure for so many kids.
>
> And third, that the moment we closed schools, we didn't immediately start planning about how to reopen them. Which is how we've landed one month or two weeks before schools open with kids, many of whom who have not had a meaningful educational experience in the spring, soaring numbers in many counties and most school districts, and schools struggling to put together some kind of a coherent plan for how to bring kids back, if at all.

NO ONE WAS IN CHARGE OF REOPENING SCHOOLS

And that's part of the problem. We didn't immediately start planning how to reopen schools because, for one thing, there was no meaningful "we."

The federal government left it up to the states. States largely passed the buck to districts. And districts were overwhelmed.

Put yourself in the position of a beleaguered school administrator for a moment. At the exact moment in the spring when she would normally begin planning for the fall, she was busy standing up emergency remote learning and emergency feeding programs amid an unprecedented, unpredictable, society-wide catastrophe.

Then over the summer, she was tasked with two entirely different and novel challenges. She had to design more robust online learning programs and simultaneously change up staffing, scheduling, cleaning, and everything in between for in-person school (formerly known as "school"). Most of the schools that offered hybrid schedules had to master a third challenge: teaching "Zoom from the room"— meaning another way to teach, another way to lesson-plan, another set of technological challenges to master. One teacher I know called it "juggling with knives."

Now bear in mind that school districts are some of the most small-*d* democratic institutions in the country. Not only did they often have to negotiate every detail of these new plans with teacher unions; parents and the general public were weighing in endlessly. They were passionate, and their voices couldn't be ignored. The Miami school board held a twenty-nine-hour Zoom meeting about reopening plans in September 2020.

Independent schools, which educate about one in ten children and have varying levels of funding, were also left to their own devices, with even less guidance than the public schools had.

By the end of the year, not surprisingly, a wave of superintendents would quit, including the chiefs of the country's three largest districts, New York, Los Angeles, and Chicago. There would also be a record number of school board recall elections, quadruple that of a normal year.

School districts are political entities, governed by elected boards. And in the end, decisions broke out primarily along partisan lines.

Study after study found that the local percentage of Trump voters was the strongest factor determining school reopening. This played out state by state and county by county. For example, one paper found Democratic landslide counties in Michigan were four times more likely to stay fully remote than their red neighbors. There was a relationship, but a much weaker one, between local COVID rates and school reopening plans.

There were related factors pushing in the same direction. COVID itself hit Black and Latinx and Native communities harder. Parents in those districts, which often lean Democratic, correctly perceived a higher risk in coming back to school, relative to white families. Families as well as teachers in many high-poverty urban districts did not trust that their crumbling school buildings could be clean, well-ventilated, safe places. Families who were white, Republican, wealthy, rural, or some combination of the above, were more likely to push for—and to get—in-person schooling.

POLARIZATION DROWNED OUT SCIENCE

The intense politicization of the pandemic response in general, and school reopening in particular, created a cacophony that made it difficult for scientific authorities to be heard.

For example, in late June 2020 the American Academy of Pediatrics issued a statement "strongly advocat[ing] that all policy considerations for the coming school year should start with a goal of having students physically present in school." The administration repeatedly cited the guidance. The AAP's president appeared at a White House roundtable with President Trump.

Educators were publicly unhappy that the statement didn't mention their safety. Less than two weeks later, the AAP was out with a new statement, cosigned by the two national teacher unions and the School Superintendents Association, emphasizing that reopening safely would take federal resources and should be guided by "science and community circumstances."

I saw this seesaw play out on an individual level with my acquaintance Christakis. He struggled with repeated invitations to appear on Fox News, where he knew his message was being twisted to serve a Republican talking point: "open schools with precautions" would be framed as "open schools at any cost."

BEHIND TEACHER RESISTANCE

Annie Tan teaches special education in Sunset Park, Brooklyn's Chinatown (she herself grew up in Manhattan's Chinatown). She's also a writer. And she's a union activist, part of the left-wing Movement of Rank and File Educators caucus within the United Federation of Teachers. UFT–NY is one of the most powerful teacher unions in the country, with two hundred thousand members.

Annie had been talking to her students about the mysterious virus in Wuhan since January 2020. "I always do this morning news segment in my class, to start the morning. As Wuhan was shutting down and quarantining, I showed my students footage of that. And the students were like, 'wow, that's like *Resident Evil*,'" the zombie apocalypse video game and movie franchise.

On March 4, a suspected coronavirus infection was reported by a New York City teacher who had recently returned from Italy. There followed a fateful period of uncertainty and mistrust that laid the groundwork for what happened in the fall. Annie said she and her colleagues were wondering, "Why are all of these establishments closed, why is Broadway closed before schools? It just felt like we were being completely ignored."

In March 2020, Mayor Bill de Blasio said CDC-approved cleaning supplies were going out to all schools and that the buildings would be deep cleaned twice a week. Annie and her colleagues "called bullshit." "They weren't hiring more staff, and the custodians had way more than enough to do. In fact, they always work overtime anyway. One of the things they said for deep cleaning was, we will wipe down all the desks every day. So we...drew in pencil on the desk to see if it would be cleaned. And it wasn't."

Many bathrooms in her school were closed, as they often were, because fixtures were broken. And there was never any soap. Annie's principal told her to tell the kids to wash their hands before coming to school and after going home. She was issued a small bottle of hand sanitizer. "So we were like, they are not taking this seriously at all. Are you kidding me?"

Negotiations with teachers over school reopening hinged on protocols about ventilation, surface disinfection, student contact hours, and average class size. But really they were about trust and respect.

I heard again and again from teachers like Tan that they didn't trust school leadership to keep them safe, because they worked in buildings where they and their students weren't taken care of.

NO TRUST, NO RESPECT

Public school educators have a unique occupational role and history in the United States, which illuminates the resistance of a vocal minority of teachers to coming back to the classroom.

New York Times education reporter Dana Goldstein's 2014 book *The Teacher Wars* is subtitled *A History of America's Most Embattled Profession*. That word "profession" goes right to what's embattled about it. Teachers' status and identity as professionals are precarious.

Teachers are college educated—many with advanced degrees—salaried, often tenured, and certified to standards maintained by peers. These characteristics define a professional.

But, beginning in the nineteenth century, teaching evolved into a female-dominated profession. Three-quarters of K–12 teachers are women still today. That's not true of most other professions; only a little over a third of doctors are women, for example. In her book, Goldstein argues that teachers in the United States have had trouble getting respect because the profession is so gender skewed. Fewer men enter the profession because it's less respected by virtue of being "women's work." The relative status of the profession has also fallen over the generations, as women have had other occupations open up to them.

With lower status comes lower pay: teachers earn about 20 percent less than other college-educated workers at similar levels of experience.

Public school teachers are also public-sector workers. Other public-sector workers are not typically considered professionals.

I'm emphasizing these contradictions because during the pandemic, occupational safety broke along status lines. College-educated professionals like me were largely able to stay home and work on a laptop, with the notable (and noble) exception of health-care professionals.

Under the brutal pressures of the pandemic, people with work-from-home privilege were in danger of developing a certain callousness. We preserved our own safety even when it put other people at risk. I struggled with the implicit calculus of ordering takeout, knowing it was cooked in a crowded kitchen, rather than risk going to the grocery store myself.

Not everyone had this luxury, the luxury to stay home and stay afraid. Falling into the broader category of essential workers were many of teachers' fellow unionized city and county employees, like bus drivers, police officers, firefighters, and sanitation workers. They showed up to work in person from day one of the pandemic. Many got sick and died. They didn't grab headlines with strike threats or protests or lawsuits—at least not until vaccine mandates came along in 2021. There wasn't a huge public debate over whether they should go to work. That's what "essential worker" meant.

There were plenty of public school employees who kept coming to work too. Like a quarter-million food service workers. Many of the nation's 350,000 custodians worked harder than they ever had in their lives to keep up with new sanitation protocols. In New York City during the height of the first surge, some school carpenters were put to work in a high school gym, building coffins.

Childcare workers—who earned less and were more likely to be people of color than were public school teachers—continued to show up in person as well. When teachers acted to delay or limit school reopening, their actions did not shield the people who, typically for low wages and no benefits, staffed alternative group childcare arrangements like learning hubs and in-home daycare centers in every city where schools stayed remote.

Patricia was in no hurry to return to the classroom herself, but she didn't think it was too risky to send her sons to group daycares. She sent her older son to Gifted Academy using barter and sweat equity to make up some of the fees. Her toddler, Patrick, went to a different daycare where she could use her city vouchers.

Patricia told me it was an easy decision. She trusted her friend more than her own employer. Garza's husband had built Plexiglas dividers to place between the children's desks. It was fewer kids than PJ would be with in the classroom.

She'd taught in pre-K classes in the DC public schools where mice ran over the children as they napped on their mats. "The schools are still dirty. The windows don't open fully. They still don't have what they need. What have you shown me any different?" she wanted to know.

MOST TEACHERS SHOWED UP

Teachers, and specifically teacher union resistance to working in person, dominated media coverage in the fall of 2020. Unions filed lawsuits. There were a few small strikes and many more strike threats from big-city unions. There were sickouts. There were protests in which teachers carried cardboard models of children's coffins.

Annie Tan was among those who changed her Twitter handle to "Annie Won't Die for DOE" (New York City's Department of Education).

This resistance helped prolong school closures, particularly in big, Democratic cities. And it arguably contributed to poor families of color being disproportionately afraid to come back to the classroom. Families trusted their teachers, and by brandishing child-sized coffins, teachers were evoking intense fear.

But this kind of militant resistance wasn't at all the typical teacher experience or viewpoint. If Burbio's data is roughly accurate, around six in ten public school teachers in the United States returned to teaching in person by October 2020 even if many of their students stayed home. And throughout the school year, more teachers returned.

Like Jeannie, they showed up even when they were scared, even when they were angry, and even when they sometimes got sick. In doing so, they acted in the roles of essential workers and public servants. Maybe they did more than we should have asked of them. They also did what their students needed.

Tan organized her colleagues to threaten a strike over safety measures. She never stopped trying to hold the city accountable for falling short in its promised safety protocols. But personally, she opted not to take a medical exemption for her asthma when schools ultimately opened in New York City, after two delays, in late September 2020. "Teachers, in our heart of hearts, were like, no, let's do this for our students. Maybe this won't be as bad as we think."

THE ROLE OF UNIONS

Advocates of open schools sometimes argued that unions led their rank and file astray by pursuing dead-ender opposition to reopening. They pointed to close ties between the two national teacher unions and the Democratic Party, ties that may have led them to lean into and exacerbate the partisan divide over the issue in the runup to the election. Dr. Jill Biden, now the First Lady, is a member of the National Education Association. Randi Weingarten, the head of the American Federation of Teachers, attacked Trump continuously on Twitter.

Putting that argument in perspective takes a little bit of recent history. Most public school teachers are in unions. But twenty-seven states have right-to-work laws, limiting union power. Teacher union power was further limited by the *Janus* Supreme Court decision in 2018. This was a case instigated and supported by part of the Republican coalition: anti-union activists whose intellectual grandfather is James McGill Buchanan, the progenitor of the anti–public school movement described in Chapter 1.

Janus found that public employees whose workplace is covered by a union contract don't have to pay dues to that union. They can be free riders. *Janus* meant unions stood to lose both members and revenue. Political scientists I spoke to at the time argued that it could also lead to unions getting more involved in politics, to prove their mettle to their members.

Teacher union power was challenged in a different way by the "Red for Ed" wave that swept the country in 2018. These were wildcat teacher strikes and protests. They happened in right-to-work states like West Virginia, Arizona, and Oklahoma. Teachers organized on social media and won concessions from state legislatures. The whole time, they enjoyed broad support from parents, even in very red states. And they did all of this largely without unions.

So when the pandemic struck, unions were on their back foot in lots of ways, but the potential for collective resistance among teachers was high.

Looking at all the factors that undermined the school reopening process in the United States, I don't see unions as the puppet master. I see them as just one group of players. The fact that teachers like Annie Tan largely went into the classroom when they were called underlines that the core intention of teachers in opposing reopening was to use their leverage to make schools safer for both themselves and their students. And perhaps, to seize the pandemic pause as a chance to reconsider just whose interests public schools had been serving in the years prior to 2020 and whether they could be made to do better.

BLACK LIVES MATTER AND SCHOOL REOPENING

The Black Lives Matter uprising of the summer of 2020 influenced the school reopening debate. Black, Latinx, and Asian American families were more reluctant to return to school in person. Teachers, who are primarily white women, pointed to the disproportionate impact of COVID-19 on Black and Brown people in arguing against opening schools.

The United Teachers of Los Angeles informally demanded that the police be defunded before schools could reopen. The acrimony in Chicago stood out, with rounds of late-night negotiations and strike threats creating whiplash for families throughout the school year, and race was never far from the conversation in a city where the public schools are only 11 percent white. The Chicago Teachers Union at one point posted, then deleted, a tweet saying the push to reopen schools was "rooted in racism, sexism and misogyny." At Highline Public Schools near Seattle, graffiti read, "Racist superintendent. Reparations now."

On the other side, the public faces of the school reopening movement tended to be white mothers. They, too, sought to frame reopening as an equity issue. Their opponents weren't buying it.

"Soccer moms suddenly profess concern for inner city kids in one breath, and prospects for college admissions for their own kids in the other, as though the stakes are the same," wrote Rashelle Chase Hibbard, an early childhood educator who is white, in an article headlined "The 'Reopen Schools Now!' Debate Is Rooted in Racism." "We see white and affluent parents leveraging the plight of historically underserved children as justification to reopen schools now, while actively excluding the communities they claim to be advocating for from the conversation."

FLORIDA VERSUS CALIFORNIA

Why was it so hard?

These decisions shouldn't have been left up to districts in the first place. They were mired in political battles. They had little relevant expertise to judge incomplete and emerging evidence. My intention here in this chapter is not to relitigate this mess or point fingers. I want to reconstruct the impact on children.

Children who had the opportunity to go to school in person full-time had a clear advantage in 2020–2021. They missed many days for quarantines, and this could add up to learning setbacks. But they had the greatest possible degree of normalcy in this very strange year. Teachers and parents reported they made progress on the learning lost in the spring, and social isolation eased, even when attending school in masks and with distancing. After controlling for gender, race, and class, research showed those who had the ability to attend high school in person during the pandemic did better academically, emotionally, and most of all socially.

Robin Nelson is a first grade teacher at Ortega Elementary in Jacksonville, Florida. The school is two-thirds low income and nearly evenly split among white, Black, and Latino students.

When I first spoke to her for NPR, a few weeks into the shutdown in March, she wept as she talked about missing her "babies." "A computer can't hug you," she said. "A computer is not your teacher."

She was back in the classroom October 1, 2020, and it was a joyful reunion. "I was so glad to have my hands on them. Computer teaching is not the same. It's just not." She was relieved to be done with the little heartbreaks of separation, like seeing students nod off on the other side of the screen. "And you can only say, hey, sweetheart, wake up! You know, you need the physical in person to do a complete job."

This was Florida, a state where the governor would attempt to ban school mask mandates in the fall of 2021. But Nelson had confidence in her school's COVID protocols in the fall of 2020. "I've got about fourteen or fifteen kids. The desks have at least one desk in between each other, so everybody has a little bit of elbow room. We have the hand sanitizer and we wear face masks." She found the kids amazingly compliant in their mask wearing, with gentle reminders. Ortega got through the whole year without any major outbreaks.

It was a lot of creativity, a lot of little adjustments. The students ate lunch in the classroom instead of the cafeteria, with a Disney movie on so they didn't talk too much. No more sharing crayons. Recess was shorter, and they couldn't mingle with other classes on the playground. In place of partner work, "where they're in each other's faces," Nelson tried to engage the whole class in discussion. They would pull down their masks and put on a face shield when they needed to practice letter sounds and see the difference between a *B* and a *D*. Having a smaller class size made it a little easier for her to give children individual attention, which helped.

Greetings were different too. They were no longer separated by a computer screen, but she still couldn't hug her students. "In previous years, I had a little poster in the hallway that says, 'How would you like to be greeted?' And it would be a high five and a hug or whatever.

So I've altered that. We do toe tapping, hip bump, elbow bump. But the kids still wait at the door anticipating what they can do to be greeted."

Most of Nelson's class came in behind on their learning, compared to previous years. She was able to catch them up quite a bit, but she estimated it could take another year to get them back on pace—which is exactly what education researchers would estimate as well.

KINDERGARTEN ON A PHONE

Across the country in California, it was a very different story. In Chapter 2, the hunger chapter, you met Serena and Elisa, her mother. Elisa immigrated to this country from Peru about ten years before the pandemic. Serena attends Buena Vista Horace Mann, a K–8 public school in San Francisco. The two speak primarily Spanish, as do most of the students in the school.

Buena Vista Horace Mann occupies a large city block in the heart of the Mission District, a gentrifying hipster neighborhood spangled with bright murals. The nineteenth-century classroom buildings surround a garden and play yard. This is a community school. That means it partners with nonprofits and city agencies to provide as many services as possible to its students. A few years ago, Buena Vista Horace Mann converted one of its gyms to become the country's first public school to host a homeless shelter for families. During COVID, the capacity was limited, but it still housed thirty families. The school raised $70,000 to help families with direct needs like diapers, medicine, and rent. For a lot of these families, the pandemic wasn't the first tough time in their lives, and it brought up a lot of fear and anxiety. "We deal with a lot of trauma," Nick Chandler, the community-school coordinator of services, told me. "We have a lot of newcomers, migrants who've experienced some sort of trauma in their home country or crossing trauma or both."

With schools closed, Serena rode with her mother on the bus to the hotel where Elisa was a housekeeper. She had gotten a laptop from the school, but it wasn't practical to bring it along with her. So Serena's experience of kindergarten was mainly on her mother's phone.

Serena's teacher was Debby Rosenthal Harris. She's originally from Guatemala, an incredibly warm and encouraging person who wears crisp cotton dresses and espadrilles to teach. She has fifteen years of experience, and she loves kindergarten. "Kindergarten is just such a wonderful, physical, tactile age. Everything in kindergarten is very, very hands on. It's just a lot of touch and play and hugging and, you know, coziness."

Harris agreed with Robin Nelson in Florida that translating that experience online was nearly impossible. But she was working day and night to accomplish the impossible. "I was a pretty dedicated teacher to begin with, but I find that I'm spending ten or twelve hours a day thinking about a way of bringing my lessons to the kids and making it engaging and creative and fun and interesting."

The morning routine ran from 9:30 to 10:00 a.m.: yoga, breathing exercises, a song or two, and letter sounds practice. In a video she sent me, she appears in front of an alphabet poster with a bright smile, pointing to a picture of a bear and saying the word for it in Spanish. "Oso, oso, o, o, o."

Virtual attendance was usually pretty good for this morning session, but it fell off for small-group instruction and the math lesson later in the day.

Serena's mother, Elisa, usually started stripping the beds around the time of the third lesson and was in a hurry to get the linens to the laundry crew. So she often wasn't able to make sure that Serena stayed logged on after the first hour.

Elisa told me in Spanish, "It's hard for her to focus. Sometimes she's distracted and not very attentive. It's difficult for me—I know it would be easier if I were sitting next to her."

Most of Harris's students, like Serena, had a passive, TV-like experience of kindergarten. By the end of the first semester, only about a fourth of them were consistently trying the assignments she posted for them. "Some of the parents are not literate, not in Spanish and sometimes not in their Indigenous language either. As much as they love their kids, they don't feel that they know how to do this. Even when I think that I'm giving a pretty simple explanation, I have parents that say, 'I'm sorry. I'm not quite sure what you mean.'"

Harris was in touch with her families frequently. They needed help with medical care, diapers, fighting an eviction. One, a single mother with three children, was selling odds and ends on the street to survive.

Harris had all the sympathy in the world for them. But to teach this way, beating her head against a stone wall, was tough on her personally also. "If I'm working hard, and no one has looked at the lesson, it's just frustrating. It almost feels disrespectful of the amount of time that we're putting into it."

This was a really common experience for teachers I talked to. When parents, students, and teachers came back together in person, it would be in mutual incomprehension that sometimes cooled into hostility. Many teachers had been working as hard as ever in their lives, entirely reinventing their jobs, dealing with immense fear and uncertainty and shifting expectations. Meanwhile, families had been struggling with the lack of in-person school or limited and inconsistent hours with repeated and unpredictable closures. Teachers were giving more, but families were receiving less.

Harris judged that without the ability to have them in person, and to immerse them in English alongside Spanish, about a quarter of her class was making no progress at all in learning to read. Writing was perhaps even worse, considering that she was used to guiding students hand over hand.

"Every year you will have five, six kids that are struggling. They come very unprepared to school. But at least they're with me all day long. And so I can support them six or seven hours a day." By December 2020, after half a year of remote teaching, she said, "I'm starting to see a lot of growth with my kids. But those four or five or six kids that are low, I'm starting to see a very big gap between them and everybody else."

Harris's observation of her class exactly tracked what international development experts told me at the beginning of the pandemic. During a natural disaster, any attempt to make up for the loss of in-person school will tend to widen existing gaps.

Another way of looking at it: in-person, free universal public school has a particular power as a social equalizer. And the lack of it multiplies inequality.

EVERYONE HAD THEIR OWN SET OF FACTS

The conversation about school reopening drew more heat than light in the fall of 2020. And as the weeks and months wore on, it didn't get better. You might think that the relative risks and safer strategies for school reopening would have become clearer over time.

But that took a while. And pro– and anti–school opening groups hardened in their positions.

Partly it was because cases were growing; it was hard to detect the signal from school reopening in the rumble of another COVID wave.

Florida, with its open schools, became a national hotspot. Later, California, with closed schools, led the ranks. New Jersey, during the time that it had the highest death rate in the nation, was a purple state with closed and open districts cheek by jowl.

Without effective and reliable contact tracing, enough testing, or other large-scale data collection, nobody had great real-time information about whether, where, and why schools in the United States were really driving the spread of COVID. There were reassuring studies from other countries, but the data was limited.

"We're driving with the headlights off, and we have kids in the car," Melinda Buntin, chair of the Department of Health Policy at Vanderbilt School of Medicine, told me for NPR in October 2020—though she still argued on balance in favor of opening schools, with precautions.

By the winter, peer-reviewed evidence from the United States showed that schools with layers of COVID precautions in place could and did operate with lower levels of infection than surrounding communities, even when that community spread was quite high. But those numbers came pretty late in the game to influence decision paths.

THERE ARE NO GOOD OPTIONS

In red counties, there were schools that opened up full-time right away, ignoring social distancing and even masking. Some teachers, like Jeannie, were scared to come to work this way. I spoke to a teacher in DeKalb County, Georgia, who took a shower and changed her clothes upon coming home every night for fear of exposing her son, who had asthma. Later in the year she left the classroom. Another teacher, in Ohio, who had a high-risk health condition, hung up a clear plastic shower curtain around her desk and shouted at students from behind her improvised isolation booth.

Open schools often had to close again, unpredictably, when cases turned up, sending home a few students, a single classroom, a school, or an entire district. Teachers reported that they struggled to get teenage boys and students with disabilities to keep masks on.

In both hybrid and full-time settings, teachers were hamstrung by the requirement to teach both remote and in-person students. Sometimes they had to do this simultaneously—shouting through a mask and a face shield to be heard by children on Zoom.

"I don't feel like I've really done a whole lot of teaching this year. And the chances of any of [my kids'] teachers feeling like they're doing a wonderful job are pretty slim," Jeannie told me. Some surveys showed that kids in hybrid fell even further behind than kids in all-remote. It was that disruptive.

The requirement to teach in both modes seemed especially galling when teachers saw that the students who needed more support, who were often students of color and low-income students, were more likely to be staying home. Annie Tan in Brooklyn had at some points three in-person students and six at home. Every night, after she went home, she would spend hours helping her virtual students.

REMOTE POSSIBILITIES—FINDING A TRUSTED ADULT

It's hard but not unheard of for students to succeed in remote learning. The key wasn't the computers or the hotspots, although those were prerequisites. It was relationships.

Students stayed connected in schools that already had support programs in place, through the commitment of individual teachers, community groups, and families and caregivers with the energy and skills to help them.

Oakland Reach, from Chapter 4, is a community organization that shifted from organizing parents to push for better schools to directly helping those parents with basic needs and education. After running a successful virtual hub over the summer, the organization kept offering families virtual tutoring with certified teachers on the weekends throughout the school year. The combination of motivated families and individual attention helped; students kept up in reading and math.

I talked to Emmanuel, who lives in Flatbush, Brooklyn, with his mother and grandmother. He had struggled academically before following in his brother's footsteps to Liberation Diploma Plus, an alternative public high school in Coney Island. The school is small and focused on giving students personalized paths to graduation.

Despite lockdown and its discontents, despite anxiety, loneliness, and depression, Emmanuel successfully finished up his high school degree at the age of twenty, in the winter of 2021. And he credited his friends and his teachers. "The school is more like a family than staff and students. We interact with each other; we talk to each other every day."

Christian is a high school student and avid baseball player who came to Florida from Puerto Rico after Hurricane Maria. His father is a plumber who had to keep working in person after lockdown. He sent Christian back to Puerto Rico to live with his mother, believing he'd be safer there.

Christian is exactly the type of student most likely to disappear from school during a closure and not be heard from again. But his high school, a large, diverse, comprehensive public school in Florida, uses BARR (Building Assets, Reducing Risks), a school-wide drop-out prevention program that has piled up reams of solid evidence and is used all over the country.

Essentially, the adults in the school get together regularly to identify which students need attention and create plans to help them. They work to build positive relationships and recognize students' strengths. "We call it the Wolf Pack Family," the hearty principal, Ed Mathews, told me.

In the spring, Christian got a Chromebook from the school and heard regularly from his bilingual mentor. He was able to keep up with his assignments in tenth grade even though he was now hundreds of miles away. He wanted to stay connected to school so he could stay on the varsity baseball squad.

ALL THE WAYS REMOTE CAN FAIL

These are the circumstances where remote went well. This book is, however, more concerned with the large percentage of children for whom it didn't go well. At all.

Buena Vista Horace Mann is an exemplary school for a high-need population. It helped underconnected families get devices and Wi-Fi. Teachers teamed up across each grade level so that students could have both whole-class and small-group instruction every day. The teachers, like Harris, stretched and innovated, did their own research, and created engaging lessons. They created and edited video and audio clips, used new software platforms, and essentially changed the entire nature of their job to adapt to this new medium, an astonishing accomplishment.

But on the other side of the screen, there were big problems.

Technical failures, of course. A nationally representative survey of families earning below the median household income—which was $67,521 in 2020—found that 53 percent of remote students experienced a learning disruption during the 2020–2021 school year because of underconnectedness. That included being unable to participate in class or complete their schoolwork because of a lack of internet access or a computer, or having to do their schoolwork on a smartphone at some point, like Serena.

Beyond technical problems, there was a more basic issue that didn't just affect lower-income students. It was about the agreement made between teacher and student. Washington Heights teacher José Luis Vilson's observation at the beginning of the pandemic held true. Remote education was not compulsory. A student could switch to another browser window or simply walk away at any time. Several parents told me that their kids spent weeks watching YouTube videos instead of class before the teacher finally alerted them. This happened even in professional families with a stay-at-home parent. Only a lucky minority of students had the combination of inner fortitude, material resources, and consistent in-person adult help (cajoling or coercion) necessary to succeed.

In October 2020 teachers and principals reported the following: First, the highest-poverty schools as well as those with the most Black and Brown students were less likely to offer in-person instruction. Second, kids were disappearing. Teachers said that they were unable to even contact one-fifth of their students, similar figures to spring 2020. For Jeannie, five out of thirty-five sixth graders weren't turning in any work. By November she'd already requested that the school consider retaining them. "They're missing a whole year." Others were dropping off her rolls, possibly going to homeschooling or charter schools.

High levels of severe chronic absence and disengagement from school persisted throughout the year. Nineteen states didn't even require daily attendance-taking in remote learning. The nonprofit Attendance Works reported a growing number of students missing more than half of the school year. In the fall of 2020, some districts reported huge increases in failing grades. In Maryland's largest school district, 36 percent of low-income freshmen failed the first marking period in English—six times higher than that same group of students the year before.

These headwinds took their toll on teachers. Four of five reported feelings of burnout. Like Harris, they were working harder than ever before, yet they were haunted by the knowledge that what they were doing still wasn't enough.

"They're reading *Bridge to Terabithia* right now and they're answering comprehension questions," Jeannie told me in the fall. "And then I have, in addition to that, a little grammar video and quizzes they complete. And I really don't think that that's quality. I mean, they need some explanation, and I know that there's a video with it, but that's a minute and thirty seconds. It probably isn't enough for a lot of those kids. A lot of our kids are low [achievers] anyway. And so, I don't think that I'm doing a great job at all."

ONLINE LEARNING AND MENTAL HEALTH

Students weren't just being obstinate. They were failing to cope because online school wasn't providing what they desperately needed. Melinda Macht Greenberg is a psychologist who works with schools in Massachusetts. "I'm seeing kids of all ages who are not able to access education from home," she tells me. "I'm hearing about the kids and the teenagers who are in bed all day and unable to function even to go and log in to their computer to join the class."

She broke down for me how online learning didn't serve basic developmental needs. "All kids need social learning. The social aspect of learning is critical not only for social skill building and motivation and emotional support, but also because kids are learning from each other. It allows people to learn and to stay motivated and engaged."

Some children can sit and read or watch videos day after day and successfully process what they've learned, maybe with a few chats with a teacher—a skill that would seem more appropriate to expect of adults. But most, says Macht Greenberg, "don't have the executive

functioning skills...to be able to work independently for long periods of time or to teach themselves information, which is why it falls
on parents and caregivers and people to support them. And without
it, it's a flat screen. And as you know, as one child said to me, I
feel like I'm doing homework all day long. There's nothing to sustain
them and it's untenable."

Remote teachers tried hard to stimulate social learning. They used
breakout rooms on Zoom to hold small-group discussions or put discussion questions in text forums. Sometimes this worked and sometimes it didn't. I dropped in on Zoom classrooms and witnessed the
vicious circle. Teachers made lesson plans that depended on student
participation; they were greeted day after day by cameras turned off
or pointed at the ceiling and silence; they defaulted to the sound of
their own voices. Some private and charter schools required students
to keep their cameras on, which helped to reinforce participation.
Many public schools worried about the invasion of privacy or violation of equity this practice could pose.

STUDENTS DIDN'T LEARN AS MUCH WHEN SCHOOLS WERE CLOSED

From the time that schools first closed in March 2020, people worried students wouldn't learn as much. But learning is hard to quan-
tify. The common way we have measured student learning in school
in the twenty-first century is standardized, multiple-choice reading
and math assessments.

As I reported in my 2015 book, *The Test*, these instruments are
cheap and efficient and can be compared easily across different con-
texts. They also have lots of drawbacks. They are narrow and shallow.
They don't address the most important learning outcomes, such as
critical thinking, collaboration, and creativity. When these tests have
high stakes attached, they've been shown to distort the curriculum
and introduce a false sense of precision to the highly individualized
process of learning. Standardized scores can be depressed if the room

is too hot, if children haven't had breakfast, or if they are reminded of their status as girls or as Black people before the exam—what is called "stereotype threat."

In the spring of 2020, mandatory state testing was suspended across the country for the first time since it was established in 2001. The pause demonstrated that these tests are inessential. But with no immediate substitute, it also created another pandemic-related data void.

Testing picked back up in the fall. Software-based learning programs in some cases collected continuous data, compiling student answers on every homework problem, quiz, and test. And Miguel Cardona, Joe Biden's education secretary, instructed all states to assess students in the spring, though states varied in how many students were able to participate.

The data was imperfect and incomplete, but it matched past experience and common sense. Students hadn't learned as much math or reading, as far as was measurable, as they would in a typical year. The students who had the least access to in-person instruction learned the least. One analysis used Hurricane Katrina as a benchmark, as I had back in March 2020. It estimated that the impact of COVID was two to four times greater. Recall that students who went through Katrina took two years on average to return to their previous academic trajectory, and many dropped out of school altogether.

Researchers feared that the true situation was even worse than these scores revealed, because some of the students who were disengaged from school—disproportionately low income, Black, and Latinx—weren't participating. Schools, other institutions, and families have hard work to do to help kids, and it's going to be over years, not months.

SERENA ISN'T DOING MUCH KINDERGARTEN

I met up with Serena, Elisa, and Serena's teacher, Debby Rosenthal Harris, outside Horace Mann one afternoon in the spring. San Francisco's schools had just opened up part-time, for the last six weeks of the year, and a small proportion of students had returned. It was a windy day, and mother and daughter were bundled up in puffer jackets. Serena was a small frowning girl with shining black hair. She ignored a pile of picture books that her teacher brought for her and asked for her mother's phone.

She wasn't doing well, her mother told me. She had one friend from preschool who she would see sometimes for playdates, and otherwise it was just the two of them. She wanted her mother's phone all the time and didn't want to play outside. She would watch cartoons on YouTube or sometimes videos on TikTok that her mother didn't understand and worried were inappropriate.

Elisa berated herself for not spending more time reading to Serena, who showed little interest in books.

> My life is very rushed. I don't have time to sit and read. I would like to sit with her and help her with her homework, help her with her classes, but I can't. I can't always keep an eye on her, so she's seeing things she shouldn't be watching.
>
> Sometimes she gets angry at me. She will push me. She says to me, "I don't love you. When am I going to go out? I'm tired of being inside."

THE FAMILIES I FOLLOWED STRUGGLED WITH REMOTE LEARNING

Every family I followed in detail during the pandemic struggled with remote learning. Dara's son Charlie had Valencia, the au pair, to make sure he was finishing his work. Hannah, her oldest, would wake up a few minutes before class and procrastinate on all her assignments until late at night. "My sleep habits are terrible," she told me.

Jonah, the eleven-year-old in San Francisco with learning disabilities and autism, found Zoom school unbearable. He could barely pay attention for more than a few minutes at a time. It got worse in the fall as he transitioned to a new middle school. Now he didn't know any of his teachers, and the classes were larger, more anonymous. "When it was still fifth grade, it was fine," he says. "The classes were like thirty minutes. I'd have my camera on. I'd go to my classes for the whole time. Now I never have my camera on and I only have to go to fifteen minutes of each class. If the class isn't fun, if I don't like my teacher, I'm not going to put the camera on." He found the teachers boring except for one or two, who played interesting videos or put the students into breakout rooms to chat with one another.

Jonah's foster brother Khamla did better. But as an English language learner, he sometimes struggled to understand the teachers over Zoom. He was too shy to ask them to repeat themselves.

PRIVATE SCHOOL ENROLLMENT DROPPED

Counterintuitively, traditional private school enrollment actually dropped during the first full school year of the pandemic. More than one hundred Catholic schools closed. This was also an economic crisis, after all, so not many families could find the spare cash for tuition. Social distancing requirements kept some private schools from increasing their capacity. Others remained remote where public schools were also remote, so the advantage of switching was small. The health commissioner in wealthy Montgomery County, a bastion of prep schools for the DC-area elite, went so far as to order private schools not to open their doors at the end of July 2020; New Jersey, California, and Milwaukee took similar steps.

VIRTUAL CHARTER SCHOOLS BOOMED

Virtual charter schools, on the other hand, boomed during the pandemic's first school year, adding tens of thousands of students. They are largely run by for-profit companies, like K12 and Connections Academy.

After their second COVID quarantine of the year, Jeannie took her daughters out of in-person school and put them in a virtual charter school. The lessons were self-paced, so she could work with them at night, after her own teaching duties were done. She had actually taught for the school before, and she considered it adequate if not amazing.

As I wrote for NPR in November 2020:

> Gary Miron, at Western Michigan University, has been doing annual watchdog reports on the virtual charter sector since 2012. He says, "Nothing changes—except that they continue to grow in the face of all the negative news, in the face of all the reports that demonstrate that they have terrible outcomes, and in the face of all the scandalous reports that investigative journalists continue to dig up."
>
> As Miron explains, corporate-run virtual schools have consistently been dogged by complaints about high student turnover, low student performance, fraud and waste. Low test scores, abysmal graduation rates and disputes about headcount have led these schools to be either shut down or placed at risk of closure in several states. Groups representing charter schools, like the National Association of Charter School Authorizers, have publicly questioned "whether virtual schools should be included in the charter school model at all," and called for stepped-up oversight and funding rules.

CITY-RUN LEARNING HUBS SERVED A FEW STUDENTS

Some districts partnered with nonprofits to create places to go for students who needed them most. New York City's Learning Bridges was one of the biggest, an extension of the emergency care it offered in the spring. It created a hundred thousand spots for children at city schools and other locations, including at least one homeless shelter for families. The YMCA, which had offered emergency childcare in the pandemic spring, ran similar programs in places including Boston; Chicago; Houston; Memphis; Huntsville and Montgomery, Alabama; La Crosse, Wisconsin; and Silicon Valley.

These efforts satisfied few. Some worried that learning hubs weren't safe; others argued that there weren't enough of them. The question arose: Why is it an acceptable risk for kids to be in classrooms with low-wage childcare workers, having a clearly inferior learning experience with their teacher on a screen, but it's not safe to open schools?

In San Francisco, Maya was able to get both Jonah and Khamla into a learning hub so she could have some much-needed peace and quiet for a few precious hours during the day. But the staff wasn't willing or able to follow Jonah's behavior plan and reward him for staying on task.

Harris, also in San Francisco, found that she was having trouble getting hub spots for her students. Many were on waiting lists until the spring. San Francisco had promised to serve an estimated number of vulnerable children in the city, such as refugees and inhabitants of homeless shelters and single-room-occupancy buildings. But from the perspective of Nick Chandler, who coordinates community services for the students at Harris's school, "This year just changed all that data. The families who were the most vulnerable in real life did not match up one to one with the way that they had that data organized." San Francisco promised six thousand spots and ultimately delivered twenty-five hundred.

RECOGNIZING THE LEARNING THAT HAPPENED AT HOME

When universal compulsory schooling paused, American childhood reverted to a shape that, if you squint, looks like the early nineteenth century. There's ten-year-old Ruby in the country, baking, knitting, caring for animals and younger siblings. There's seven-year-old Habersham in the city, making himself useful for a few dollars. Four-year-old Serena, tagging along to her mother's workplace. Eleven-year-old Charlie in his stately townhouse, being shepherded through his lessons by a young governess.

Most of this chapter—most of this book—is focused on how terrible, inequitable, and infuriatingly unnecessary it was to have the viable operations of our children's essential public welfare system suspended for so long.

Still.

While no one would have chosen it, it's also true that with the bell jar of compulsory education lifted, some fresh air and possibilities came into children's lives, however dire the circumstances.

Children learn whenever they're awake, and the pandemic offered an opportunity for families to explore what that meant.

Marjorie Faulstich Orellana, at UCLA, is an ethnographer of education who helps illuminate strengths where others see only disadvantage. During the pandemic her research team followed thirty-three families in the United States who were as diverse as they could find—newcomers from Central America and Asia, living in both rural and urban areas across ten different states. She asked them what they were doing at home. They told her about creating nightly gratitude rituals and holding family councils, grandmothers teaching grandchildren how to make Oaxacan *mole*, taking neighborhood walks together.

"Some young people—across race/ethnicity and social class—are thriving, freed from the drudgery of school," Orellana writes.

Children pursued their own interests, and not just in wealthy families. They picked up hobbies and crafts. They used YouTube to learn about whatever took their fancy. They explored and created worlds in Minecraft and Roblox. The platform Outschool exploded in use during the pandemic; it offered live video classes designed to cater to children's obsessions, from frogs to fairies.

The great loss, in Orellana's view, was that schools rarely were equipped to collaborate with families in these explorations. They remained beholden to external metrics, like grade-level standardized tests in math and reading. Assignments piled up that had little relevance to students' interests and that imposed on families' time and rhythms together. Parents hated to be thrust into the role of taskmaster, the least rewarding face of teaching.

To be fair, it's not like teachers had spent their summers at some wonderful, relaxing pedagogical-theory retreat, sitting lakeside and reimagining a student-led, home-based curriculum for this new pandemic era. They were scrambling under constantly changing and intensely difficult conditions.

"I certainly don't want to say this is fine," Orellana tells me. "I mean, the impact is tremendous and it's very uneven who's being affected. It's just—really powerful lessons are being learned in every single household from experiencing this pandemic and from all the adjustments families have had to make to live and learn together during this time."

Some families took their children out of school altogether. And some students dropped out. Homeschooling apparently doubled in the fall of 2020, to 11 percent of households with school-aged children, according to the Census Bureau, although there was some confusion over whether that number included folks who were confused by the question and were simply supervising remote learning.

There was also a public-school enrollment drop outright, of about 3 percent, driven by kindergarten enrollment and also concentrated in largely Black and Hispanic urban districts. Kindergarten is not compulsory in most cases, so families can sit the year out without any red tape or other penalties. But the loss of kindergarten can set students back for years to come, especially if they come from homes without a lot of time spent reading in English.

"Pandemic pods" such as the one Dara started received a lot of media attention. Dara directed the remodel of her basement into a classroom; recruited, interviewed, and hired a certified teacher; and organized eight classmates from Sammy's public school to attend. They dialed into the public school's Zoom lessons every day and enjoyed hands-on science experiments and picnics in Prospect Park.

In the sense of forming a stable social group so your child could see others and perhaps share childcare, surveys found about a third of all families were "podding" in the fall of 2020. At the level Dara was able to do it, actually hiring a teacher, it was the choice of a privileged few, perhaps 4 or 5 percent.

Once again, TANGO (There Are No Good Options) was the slogan for education in the fall of 2020. There were few outright winners in the school reopening saga. But if they knew where to look, some parents glimpsed a better learning world for their kids. If, and only if, they were willing and able to help construct it themselves.

One of the brighter examples of the path less traveled was my friend Larkin, an artist, musician, and single mother of nine-year-old Otis. Otis has autism and is highly gifted and sensitive. Online learning was a bust, so they fixed up a Sprinter van and drove from New York City to California, with their cat riding shotgun, camping and hiking along the way.

9 MENTAL HEALTH

The end of the pandemic is in sight.

> —Trump, a few hours before testing positive
> for coronavirus, along with the First Lady and
> more than a dozen staff and aides, October 2, 2020

> *October 6, 2020, US death toll reaches 210,000*

It was June 2020 when I got the first email out of the blue from a mental health professional who works with young people. Psychologist Lisa Damour wanted me to know that "the kids are not all right."

These emails kept coming all year.

Eight months later, in March 2021, Elisa Nebolsine, another practitioner, wrote:

> I wonder if I could respectfully suggest a story idea—one that is keeping me up at night—about the effects of the pandemic on kids and teens. I live and work in the DC Metro area, and we are closing in on one year of no in-person school for kids. As you know from your extensive work on kids, teens, education and parenting, the developing brain seeks and needs novelty and experience to reach its potential.
>
> We, through the best of intentions, have limited that for kids, and asked them to hit the pause button on their development.

Unfortunately, we both know that development doesn't work like that.

In my practice, I am seeing more depression and more significant depression than I have seen in 25 years of clinical work. My colleagues see the same. We are all struggling with too-big case loads of kids who are seriously in pain. I truly have never seen anything like this, and it is overwhelming.

This chapter concerns COVID and children's mental health. It could have come at any point in the book. But there is some evidence of a tipping point after we passed six solid months of the pandemic, after we started to leave the relatively lower case numbers of the summer behind, and after it really set in for young people that another disrupted school year was ahead.

The pandemic hit children differently at different ages. The youngest children acted out in response to their caregivers' stresses. When the pandemic hit, clinics that treat children under five saw increases in sleeping problems, nightmares, physical aggression, and regression behaviors like bed-wetting.

Elementary-school-age children suffered from the loss of daily routines, fear, uncertainty, and loneliness. Manifestations included anxiety, OCD, eating disorders, and suicidal thoughts.

Teenagers were dealing with something more existential. The adolescent brain craves risk, status, and accomplishment. Teens have an acute developmental need to experience new things, try hard things, and do things on their own. If they're lucky they find these outlets through friendships, school, sports, and other activities; otherwise, it might be drugs, sex, car crashes, and other bad decisions. They also are starting to set goals and look forward to the future. But they still default to short-term thinking.

The pandemic confined millions of teens to a deadening daily routine, under the thumb of anxious parents with little scope for independent action and a clouded path forward.

A depressed fifteen-year-old in Alexandria, Virginia, E., compared lockdown to solitary confinement. "Your brain is still developing, and this is like a time when you need to be out of the house and you need to be like seeing people and you need to be forming friendships."

And what's worse? She told me for NPR: "Everything is hard because there's no end to it. You know, you look at the news and it's like, we're not going to get back to concerts or school events until 2024. And I'm not even going to be in high school at that point. So it just is really sad to see what was supposed to be the best years of your life, like, go down the tubes."

In October 2020, the American Psychological Association found the young were the most stressed of any age group. Half of all teenagers said the pandemic made planning for the future feel impossible. Similarly, in September 2020, over half of eleven- to seventeen-year-olds reported having thoughts of suicide or self-harm most of the time over the previous two weeks. The youngest people in the survey were reporting more such thoughts than any other group of respondents, and more than in previous years.

This chapter discusses suicide. Suicide is preventable. Conditions like depression, anxiety, OCD, and eating disorders are treatable. Talking about mental health dispels shame and stigma. All of the children in this chapter got help. There is hope in these stories.

AVERY'S BIRTHDAY PARTY IS CANCELED

Avery is the older daughter of two tech industry professionals in Silicon Valley. She turned five years old at the beginning of lockdown. Her birthday party was canceled.

Avery is smart, highly verbal, and had shown some social anxiety in the year before the pandemic, like not wanting to climb on the play structure if kids she didn't know were there. Her mother, Sloane, said she was recovering from postpartum depression around the same time, after Avery's little sister, Hollis, was born.

In the first few months of lockdown, Sloane and her husband took advantage of generous employer leave policies. They traded off so one of them was always devoted to the kids full-time. They didn't have serious struggles over household work or money.

Nevertheless, Sloane worried that her and her husband's nervousness was rubbing off on the kids. "We try to be careful with the kids. But, we both have some anxious and depressive tendencies, and we're around each other 24/7. I'm sure that we occasionally are modeling things that aren't great."

Avery missed her friends at school, her routine, and her grandmother, who used to visit regularly. She missed little fun moments, like going for bubble tea with her mom. As the weeks dragged on, she started to talk in ways that, her mother says, "were really freaking me out."

One day, when she was playing on the stairs,

I asked her to be safe. And she got indignant and she was like, "Why? It's my choice if I fall and kill myself."

And then another day, I was running an errand to the post office and she wanted to come with me. I told her no. And she's like, "Why? I don't care if I die."

And I was like, "Can you tell me more about that, please?" And she's like, "Well, you have an extra kid, and Hollis is a good kid and I'm a bad kid."

OLIVER STOPS EATING

Beth and her husband both teach high school in Jersey City, New Jersey. Oliver is the middle of their three children.

In the early weeks of lockdown, virtual teaching kept Beth and her husband working from 5:00 a.m. until well past midnight every night. Some of her students were working and taking care of younger siblings. She told me how one of her students gradually dropped off the radar. When she tracked him down, he started crying and told her he was suicidal.

Beth and her husband also had to manage their own three kids in online school. Oliver was in kindergarten, and sometimes he'd be up until bedtime catching up on the work that he wasn't able to focus on during the day. "My middle son needs the schedule to keep him regulated. He also missed his friends. He missed normality. And he was scared. He was always talking about coronavirus, [that] kids are getting sick and people are going to die."

As the 2020 school year neared its end, it seemed to sink in for Oliver that "he wasn't ever going to go back to school and see his friends. I think that's what kind of tipped him to that point."

The point where he stopped eating. "Anorexia's not the right word. It was like a Gandhi hunger strike."

His parents wondered whether the sudden drop in appetite was because Oliver was less active during lockdown. They thought maybe his newly growing-in adult teeth were bothering him. They tempted him with buttered toast made with the softest white bread, which was usually off-limits in their house. But the next time she went back to the store, that brand was all gone, and Beth was too afraid of COVID to drive around to different stores looking for it.

"Then we were like, forcing him. 'You cannot leave this table until you eat.'"

This went on for weeks. They were so busy, so distracted, so overwhelmed. "So my husband and I, sometimes for dinnertime, we would plop them in front of the TV or we would make them sit at the table with us—because we were working. But then he got really clever and he started spitting into a napkin."

One night she said to her husband, "I feel like he's not eating."

"And he said, 'No, he is eating.' And then we look through the garbage. And there was this whole day of, like, spitting out." Bites of food hidden in wadded-up napkins—waffles, sandwiches, broccoli. As she told me this, Beth started to cry.

Oliver's face had grown thin. His brown eyes loomed. He was pale, and bruises showed up easily on his skin. Like Avery, he expressed suicidal thoughts. "He was, like, just lying in his bed," says his mother. "My baby. Saying he would just rather die, over and over and over again."

There seems to have been a growth in depression and "suicidal ideation"—thoughts of suicide put into words—among young people, even very young children like Oliver and Avery, during the pandemic.

Parents struggle with hearing such statements. They don't know how literally to take them. Beth thought to herself, "No you don't [want to die]. You don't even know what death is. You just want to see your friends."

One recent study showed that even as young as four years old, depressed children who talk about dying have a clearer understanding of the violence and permanence of death than their peers. This suggests that these comments are to be taken just as seriously in young children as they are in adolescents and adults.

Historically, children younger than puberty have been very unlikely to complete suicide. This is still true. But the incidence of suicide in the age group of ten to fourteen years old, while still very low, tripled from 2007 to the start of the pandemic. Among older teenagers, fifteen to nineteen, suicide rates increased in the 2000s and 2010s as well, after declining in the 1990s, and it became the second leading cause of death in this age group.

Like so many circumstances involving suffering children, the topic of their mental health causes adults so much distress that we compound the problem by ignoring it. There isn't enough research or public discussion of children's mental health. And there also aren't enough practitioners to take care of them. Children who are abused or witness community or domestic violence are more likely to become severely depressed and suicidal. But Oliver's and Avery's stories show that it can happen to any child, particularly in a society-wide crisis like the pandemic.

DAYANA DOESN'T LEAVE HER ROOM

Dayana grew up in Caracas, the capital of Venezuela. "My house was surrounded by a garden full of orchids and a parrot who called out my name," she wrote for a student publication. "I often sat there and thought, I wouldn't want to live anywhere else."

Venezuela's crisis came in 2017. The family stood in six-hour lines to buy food. Hospitals and clinics ran out of medicine. There were blackouts and outbreaks of diseases like malaria.

Her parents sat her and her little brother down and told them it was time to leave. She was fifteen years old.

They moved to the Flatbush section of Brooklyn, near Eastern Parkway. Her father got a construction job, and her mother worked doing hair, then in a store. Dayana enrolled in Brooklyn International School, a public high school with English language learners from all over the world. She joined clubs, played soccer, and loved music and writing. She was looking forward to the senior class trip to Washington, DC.

She also battled anxiety and claustrophobia—having panic attacks in an elevator that got stuck once at school, and on the subway. She saw the school psychologist and learned breathing exercises to help manage her emotions.

Then came lockdown. Her whole family was afraid. Her father and mother stopped going to work. Dayana didn't leave her apartment at all for over a month. Neither did her little brother.

"Everybody's different. Some people can do it. But I think that if I go out, something is going to happen."

Her anxiety was worse than ever. She wasn't sleeping much. She stayed up late every night chatting with her friends or watching YouTube. For her friends back home in Venezuela, things were even worse than in New York. She stopped following the news after a while because it was too scary. She would sit up in bed for her school's roll call on the computer, and then go back to sleep.

Gradually she filled the wall behind her bed with detailed pencil drawings on paper. One of them shows a girl sitting on her bed with arms crossed, looking out the window. There is a padlock on the frame. "Global Pandemic! Schools Cancelled!" it says.

Dayana started talking to the school psychologist over Google Meet. In the morning and the evening she played nature sounds and did breathing exercises. And she wrote, publishing pieces in a student journal. "Writing poetry and stories have been a great help to me. During this time I wrote a phrase that keeps me inspired: 'There is no greater loneliness than the one we impose on ourselves.' Sometimes we are not alone, support from important people is there if we seek it, but we often make ourselves believe that we are alone. That's when anxieties and fear can grow."

EBONY IS OVERWHELMED

Ebony grew up in New Orleans East, a middle-class Black neighborhood, and left home as a young teenager.

Out on her own, "I kind of got the way of the world, like capitalism, how money works. I wasn't oblivious to everything that was going on around me. So I know for a fact the only way out of this mess is school and work. So that's what I want—to go to school and get out as fast as I can so I can be into my career. I want to be a pediatrician."

She enrolled in a second-chance alternative high school called the Net and was on track for early graduation from high school at age sixteen. "I was the girl that was always at the top of the class. Always had the highest scores." Her school principal agrees that she is an exceptional young woman—a star.

When she talks to me over video for NPR, she's made up glamorously—she calls herself a "beauty guru"—and vibrating with nervous energy. She scoots around the frame on a wheeled office chair, clapping to punctuate her sentences.

When lockdown started, Ebony was living with her best friend. The house had a total of fourteen people, including half a dozen children younger than Ebony. She was "auntie" to them all and had helped raise them from babies, she tells me. Many of the adults were working, so Ebony was the point person a lot of the time. In the morning she was cooking breakfast and juggling Zoom passwords to get everyone on their online school. "It was really confusing. A few of them stopped going to school for a little while."

I've talked about the unequal division of domestic labor by gender and how it compounded the stress of the pandemic for mothers. This pattern repeated itself with girls. Across the country and around the world, girls were tasked with caregiving, at the cost of their own schoolwork and sometimes their sanity.

In the past Ebony has struggled with depression and anxiety, including social anxiety. "It takes me a lot to even want to be around people," she says. "So imagine we have all these people in one household with all the noise and just—it's too loud. It was very overwhelming for me. I just, I would go crazy. So I decided I would go spend a few days at the hospital."

In June 2020 Ebony was hospitalized for acute anxiety. She had overcome so much in her life, but the increased responsibilities and worries of the pandemic had brought her past her limits.

ROB TELLS A FRIEND A SECRET

Over a ninth grade year spent mostly in his room, Rob, Jeannie's middle child, was growing into a metalhead. He liked anime, first-person shooter games, the family pets, and Slipknot, a band that wears horror-movie masks. Up late at night and inside most of the day, Rob had an increasingly bleak outlook.

His mother didn't trust him to see his friends safely. Once in the fall he went on a sleepover, but Jeannie found out afterward that the friend had switched to in-person from virtual school, and that bothered her. A second time she agreed to let him go hiking, and it turned out to be a big group of kids. "I should have asked more questions. When he came home, he said there were a lot of people there and he started naming all these people. And I said, well, did you wear your mask? And he said, no, I was outside. So for several days, I was very worried about that because then I was hearing that certain ones were going into quarantine who were in that group....And so I told him from now on, he's just not going to get to go anywhere until there's a vaccine."

Julian had his job at Sonic. The twins and Ruby had gymnastics and piano. Rob didn't have anything getting him out of the house regularly or with people his own age. He also didn't have as many household responsibilities as his little sister. For a while his mother tasked him with cooking dinner for the family, from a Christian-influenced diet cookbook called *Trim Healthy Mama*. But he was diffident about it, and she gave up. She often called him lazy.

Jeannie thought her kids were doing fine, and that Rob was going through normal puberty struggles just like his older brothers had. "I've been going around telling people, oh, my kids have been doing so great this year. They've been home and they have each other and they don't need anybody else."

And then, in March 2021, "I get called to the junior high counselor's office"—in the school where Jeannie teaches.

I was thinking, like, OK, so I have done something terrible and I'm going to get fired because I've upset a child and didn't even have a clue because I have so many traumatized kids. They wouldn't tell me why I was being called to the office and I was about to just, like, die from that walk, not knowing what I was going into.

So I get over there and they tell me that Rob—he's not a student there this year, but he had said some things to one of his friends who is, and that the mother of that student went to the principal, and he had made, like, suicidal comments.

I went home and talked to him. And the next day I took him to be evaluated and it was decided that he wasn't a threat to himself. So they recommended counseling.

JONAH HAS A HARD TIME BACK AT SCHOOL

In the fall of 2021, Jonah started his third new school in three years. Pre-pandemic, he was an elementary school student with one teacher and a group of classmates he'd been with for years. Now he was a seventh grader with class changes, a locker, and lots of different teachers. There was a staffing crisis at his school, as there was in schools across the country that semester, and so much turnover on the special education team that his individual education plan was, according to Maya, hardly being followed. Being at home had been awful. But being back in the classroom was stressful and overwhelming, and he hated how far behind he felt. He was biking to school, and one day he simply turned around and came back, hanging out in the driveway for hours before his parents figured it out. He was hitting his stepfather. Throwing paint on the wall. And worse.

"Since he's been in kindergarten, when Jonah feels bad about himself, he's talked about killing himself," Maya tells me. "So that's not new. But in the last couple weeks, he started putting things around his neck and experimenting. And then about a week and a half ago now, he put a cord around his neck until he turned purple and I had to take it off of him." Maya was on a call with the hospital managing her sick mother's care at the time. She brought Jonah in for observation. She was very worried. It took months to get him treatment.

A RUNAWAY COMES TO NEW YORK CITY

I spoke to a medical resident doing an adolescent psychiatric rotation in the emergency room of a private hospital on the Upper East Side of New York.

One story he told illustrates the compounding effects of the pandemic:

There was this kid who ran away from home, from Baltimore. When I took her history, she said that ever since COVID hit, her parents are working from home. Her parents are extremely agitated and are on their edge and they can't tolerate each other. "They take their frustration, their job frustrations out on me. They have been physically abusing me and I've just had it with them."

So she ran away from Baltimore, took a train to come to New York, checked into a hotel with the intent to jump off of the roof. As you can imagine, when a hotel sees, like, a fourteen-year-old trying to check into a room by themselves, the hotel is not stupid. They understand something's wrong. NYPD showed up and brought the kid to us.

Aside from the ones brought in by the police, the young people in his ER were primarily white, affluent private school students. Kids with ADHD diagnoses came in almost manic, an effect attributed to too much screen time and disrupted sleep. There was cutting. A lot of marijuana use.

The resident treated one teenager who developed an eating disorder.

She has a history of depression and anxiety with some cutting in the past. She started seeing herself on Zoom much more than she had ever seen herself in a mirror. And then she hated how she looked and her depression worsened. And she started comparing herself to how the other people in her Zoom room were looking—so beautiful, so put together, their homes were so nice. So essentially she was like, you know, I have no control over how my room looks, but I do have control over my diet. She just stopped eating. She's lost over sixty pounds in a month and a half. And she's like, you know, some days I don't eat more than one hundred calories a day. And I still think I look so ugly and I look fat and everyone else looks so nice.

Along with depression, anxiety, and ADHD, some researchers found an increase in the severity of OCD and eating disorders among young people during the pandemic.

THE ROLE OF SCREENS IN TEEN MENTAL HEALTH

For many years before the pandemic, research and speculation have grown about the connection among smartphones, social media, video games, and teenage mental health. During the pandemic, screen use surged. How could this have affected children's mental well-being?

The answer is complicated because screen use is complicated. Some of it was arguably helpful for children. For example, social gaming offered many children a way to connect with their friends. Roblox, a gaming platform dominated by children under twelve, saw 161 percent more cash during the pandemic compared to the year before. In 2021, the largest long-term study of brain development and child health in the United States, the Adolescent Brain Cognitive Development (ABCD) study, reported a correlation between screen use, particularly video games, and children having more friends. Researchers concluded that "increased screen time is unlikely to be directly harmful."

In 2018 I published a book called *The Art of Screen Time*, which looks critically at the research on media and developing brains. Precisely because screen use is so ubiquitous, it's hard to prove any causal connection between media use patterns and any mental health outcome, bad or good. One of the more compelling hypotheses I've seen is that the relationship is bidirectional.

When you look across populations, as in the ABCD study, correlations are small. But young people with preexisting tendencies or risk factors related to anxiety and depression may be more likely to overuse technology, and to use it in ways that make their moods worse. During the pandemic, of course, young people had little choice but to spend more time logged on and less time doing activities that can help with depression, like moving their bodies.

One connection is clearly supported by evidence: screen use after dark can disrupt sleep, and poor sleep can contribute to mental health problems. The loss of daily routines messed up sleep patterns for many children and teenagers during the pandemic. There were teens like E., who compared her life to solitary confinement—a world seemingly shrunk to a circuit of bed, laptop, and phone. "I never stayed up super late pre-pandemic, but now I stay up so late. For no reason! I heard about this thing, it's like revenge sleep procrastination—like you don't have any freedom during the day, so, like, you take back your freedom by staying up all night and, like, doing your hobbies and stuff like that. And I feel like that kind of describes me and that describes a lot of my friends too."

LGBTQ YOUTH WERE VULNERABLE BUT ALSO RESILIENT

LGBTQ youth encounter bullying, homophobia, and transphobia at school and in the community. Many also lack family support and acceptance. During the pandemic some were trapped at home with unsupportive family members.

The Trevor Project surveys thirteen- to twenty-four-year-old LGBTQ youth on their mental health annually. Seven in ten described their mental health as "poor" most of the time or always during the pandemic. Only one in three said their homes were affirming. The percentage reporting suicidal thoughts was more or less stable from 2019, at a very high four in ten.

Practitioners who specialize in treating this community told me the pandemic was actually something of a mixed bag. Some teenagers are able to be out at school but not at home. With lockdown, that freedom went away. Some reported that watching themselves on Zoom hour after hour could magnify their sense of gender dysphoria—their image not matching how they felt inside.

At fifteen, before the pandemic, E. in Virginia came out as a lesbian. Her classmates weren't particularly supportive. During the pandemic, she could choose which classmates she had contact with. "I was able to have some power in the relationship." However, she says, "a lot of people my age lost all of their friends during the pandemic, including myself. I lost a lot of friends."

On the positive side, LGBTQ youth have for decades been creative in using technology to build support networks. And for those who had support at home, the time in relative isolation could be clarifying and affirming.

Renee Reopell, a therapist who focuses on queer, transgender, and nonbinary youth, told me some of the teens they cared for made progress toward coming out from the safety of home. These teens could spend time focusing on how they felt inside, without worrying about the judgment of classmates or even strangers on the street. Reopell started to get many more incoming requests for treatment. And as operating rooms opened up, they saw a rush in desire for gender-affirming surgeries as well.

THERE IS A ROAD BACK

The young people whose families I talked to all improved.

Avery improved when her family decided to "pod" with another family so she could play with a friend her own age.

Oliver's family found a teletherapist. He started eating again right away. His parents put him on a travel soccer team starting in the summer of 2020, so he could play with friends in person at least three times a week. His mom did notice some restricted eating creeping back as a stress response, especially during the winter COVID surges. But thanks to the therapist, the family had a good set of tools to help.

They completely overhauled the family's approach to eating. Whether it's at a family barbecue or at snack time at soccer practice, the family follows strict guidelines. No "clean your plate," no "vegetables, then dessert." They offer a variety of food and try to keep the pressure off.

After her hospitalization in June 2020, Ebony moved back in with her mother, where things were quieter and calmer. By the spring of 2021, she had caught up in her studies and was back on track to graduate early. Her school was already designed to be supportive and flexible, with "credit recovery" available if you fail a class. She had an internship at a farm in a city park where youth grow vegetables for people in need. School was coming back in person, so she could see friends and caring adults again.

The school where Jeannie works in small-town Oklahoma connected Rob to a therapist who lived in a nearby town. They met weekly over Zoom, and Rob was also able to text her when he needed help. He turned his grades around. By the summer he was feeling much better.

WHO WASN'T HEARD

All the stories I've told so far have one thing in common: We know about them. Because these children talked to someone. They had family and other adults who listened, and access to professional help.

For every child we hear about, there must be many more who didn't get help. They were too young to verbalize their distress. Their families were in over their heads. They couldn't find a clinician who spoke their first language. They asked for help but got stuck on a waiting list.

Habersham, the seven-year-old in St. Louis who was shot in an abandoned building, would certainly have benefited from therapy. After the shooting he became obsessed with guns, asking for a new toy gun every time they went to Goodwill. "I don't want to hurt anyone, Momma. I just want to get it to protect our family," he would say. "I don't really know what to do with him," she said.

So would Serena, the kindergartner in San Francisco who was so lonely and so angry at her mother, Elisa, the hotel housekeeper who was struggling just to keep her fed.

Mental health services are inadequate and inequitable for everyone in the United States, especially for children. Children's and adolescents' needs in particular were rising for more than a decade before the pandemic.

In 2019 there were just eighty-three hundred practicing child and adolescent psychiatrists in the United States for an estimated fifteen million children and adolescents who could have used their help.

Psychiatric treatments in general have relatively low reimbursement rates from Medicare and private insurers alike, and there are high rates of burnout and turnover in the profession. It was common before the pandemic for children and teens in crisis to wait in the emergency room for days for a proper placement. The American Academy of Child and Adolescent Psychiatry says that children with the most serious and debilitating diagnoses on average wait several *years* for appropriate treatment. It's estimated about two-thirds of children and youth who need treatment have no access to it.

DELINQUENTS, DEFECTIVES, AND THE DESTITUTE

The reasons are historical. Child psychiatry is a neglected specialty. And the origins of mental health services for children are tangled with the origins and contemporary workings of the archipelago of family surveillance, separation, and punishment described in Chapter 6.

In 1899 Illinois founded the nation's first juvenile court. The women who were board members of Hull House, the Chicago settlement house that provided childcare and was instrumental in the founding of the federal Children's Bureau, were shocked at the revelation of so much "criminality" among teenagers. They raised money to open the nation's first "juvenile psychopathic institute" in 1909. Its director, William Healy, a physician and neurologist, employed teams of psychiatrists, psychologists, and social workers.

Beginning in 1922, a charity called the Commonwealth Fund followed Healy's template and established community-based "child guidance programs" around the United States. They were primarily directed at young people who had come to the attention of the courts in one way or another. Schools also made referrals. These programs offered both treatment to children and "scientific" child-rearing advice to mothers. In this era, psychiatry often blamed mothers if their child deviated from the norm. One of the most notorious examples is Leo Kanner's 1940s theory that autism was caused by cold, emotionally withholding "refrigerator mothers."

Many prominent early voices in the field, such as Kanner and Anna Freud, were Europeans, women, or both. So the field grew on the margins of the US male-dominated medical establishment. Child psychiatry didn't become an official medical subspecialty until 1959. And it still attracts proportionately less research funding compared to adult psychiatry.

In 1969, 1978, 1983, 1990, and 2001, major government reports found that provision for youth mental health was inadequate and inequitable. The same is still true today. States don't usually have separate mental health agencies for children, so children compete with adults for scarce resources. These include dedicated inpatient beds, which number in the dozens, not hundreds, in major cities and are rarer in rural areas.

Most children find mental health care either through their pediatricians or through school. But a 2019 report by the ACLU found that 90 percent of public school students have insufficient access to mental health professionals at school because of staffing gaps.

On the one hand, the close historical ties among youth mental health, schools, juvenile courts, and the foster care system ensure a focus on the social determinants of mental health. On the other hand, we are still pathologizing poverty and sometimes criminalizing distress. For example, one in four children in foster care is prescribed psychiatric medication, often multiple medications, for years, and in many cases without being monitored adequately. Even accounting for the trauma of these children's life experiences, the dramatic overreliance on medication rather other forms of treatment has led to calls for reform.

PROVIDERS WERE ALREADY AT CAPACITY

During the pandemic, children had less access to mental health care than ever. They weren't going to the doctor. They weren't going to school.

Psychiatric beds were sometimes repurposed for COVID patients, or capacity was restricted because of social distancing.

Nick Chandler at Buena Vista Horace Mann says that a six-month wait list was par for the course, especially for clinicians who spoke Spanish. He says that families like Serena's, who are stressed about basic needs like food and shelter, almost invariably have mental health needs as well.

Five-year-old Avery's parents—affluent people with excellent insurance living in an area chockablock with educated professionals—had trouble finding her a therapist. "My insurance provider doesn't cover treatment for children her age. They referred me to a different provider," Sloane says. "And that provider gave me a list of therapists, and when I started looking them up, many of those don't treat children her age either. The one clinic that does, they weren't accepting new patients."

When I asked Brian Chu, director of the youth anxiety and depression clinic at Rutgers University, whether demand for services had gone up during the pandemic, he said there was no way of knowing. "Admissions haven't gone up, because we are always at capacity."

Melinda Macht Greenberg, a clinical, developmental, and school psychologist, is yet another practitioner who cold-called me to tell me about COVID's awful mental health impact on teenagers. She describes a revolving-door effect where she worked in Massachusetts. "Young people are in emergency rooms waiting for psychiatric beds at a much higher level than we've seen. They go to an emergency room. They eventually go into a psychiatric inpatient unit, but then they're discharged home because there aren't enough stepdown programs available, and then they go into crisis again."

COVID restrictions on visitation in locked-down wards also could make it harder for kids to get better. They couldn't see their families while they recovered.

LONG-TERM IMPACT

Experts expect to see the pandemic cast a shadow on mental health across the population for a decade or two to come, including on children who were in utero while their mothers experienced the stress of lockdown.

Lia Fernald, a professor in the School of Public Health at UC Berkeley, tells me, "When you read some child development theory, it's all about how resilient kids are. I read those things. I feel encouraged. And then I also think, their brains are being wired at this moment. And how is this not going to have longer-term effects?"

"I still think kids are pretty resilient, but I think the pandemic has had a real impact," the resident in the adolescent ER tells me. "Yes, I can stabilize your suicidal ideation, but I have no idea how this is going to impact your five-year mental health outcome. And I'm worried that it really will."

SOME FAMILIES HAVE MORE ACCESS TO MENTAL HEALTH CARE NOW

Some of the families and professionals I talked to were more optimistic than that. Beth said that she was grateful that her son's anxious and compulsive tendencies, which she believed he'd always had in some form, were out in the open. They caught it early and found a good therapist; they plan to keep working with her as Oliver grows up.

Lisa Damour, the adolescent psychologist who first contacted me to raise the alarm, said that a lasting benefit of the pandemic is that insurance companies changed their rules to allow much more access to teletherapy. This is helpful in rural areas and for families who lack cars. And Damour, like other practitioners, found that they sometimes got to know young clients better over video chat. They were more comfortable when they could talk to their therapists from their bedrooms.

However, teens whose families weren't as supportive lacked the privacy effective therapy requires. The ER resident told me about one teen whose parent hovered outside the door and objected if they touched on the subject of sexual orientation.

SCHOOL CLOSURES ARE STRESSFUL—BUT SO IS SCHOOL

Tyler Black, a child and adolescent psychiatrist, teaches at the University of British Columbia in western Canada. His was one voice taking stock of the data and arguments around children's mental health, and challenging the idea that merely reopening school buildings would be a quick fix.

To the contrary, Black says, in normal times school is a major source of psychological stress for the patients he treats. "I work as an emergency psychiatrist at a hospital. Summer months, I'm bored and winter months, I'm not. It could be a failed test. It could be social pressures. It could be coming out at school. It could be bullying. Whatever it is, [school] brings with it a host of psychiatric emergencies." The cessation of not only in-person school but the pressure to achieve could have benefited many vulnerable kids, he argues.

Black suggested that what looked like a massive swarm of new mental pain and suffering among teenagers was more akin to flipping on the light switch in the kitchen in the middle of the night and seeing a horde of cockroaches. The problem has been real and pervasive for a long time—we grownups just suddenly saw it. For example, he brought up eating disorders. Treatment center admissions for eating disorders in teenagers went up during the pandemic. "Kids were home and not able to do things," he says. "So is it that the disorder is increased? Or is it that the parents were able to see their kids' disordered behaviors more and get help for them?"

A SURPRISE IN THE STATISTICS

At the end of 2020, contrary to expectations, suicides actually declined across the population in the United States by a total of 5 percent.

In Canada, which has a robust social safety net already in place and experienced far less political polarization and social upheaval than the United States during the pandemic, suicides dropped an incredible 37 percent in the same period.

But if you look just at children, it was a darker story. On average, among children and teenagers in both countries, there was no decline in suicides.

And concealed within that broader average, for young people of color, the pandemic was especially deadly in this way. Black people aged fifteen to thirty-four and Latinx people twenty-five to thirty-four in the United States saw double-digit *increases* in suicides.

In Southern California, which had some of the longest school shutdowns in the country, suicides among adults dropped by 10 percent in 2020. Among minors, they went the opposite way, climbing by 19 percent.

This information is a bit of a Rorschach blot. Suicidologists talk about a "pull-together," or social cohesion, effect that can reduce suicides during natural disasters or war. It's possible that while this worked for adults, it wasn't strong enough to counteract all the factors we've been discussing in this chapter that harmed teens' mental health.

Black says the mental health establishment should be humbled by how little it actually knows about suicide. "Most people who die by suicide die on their first attempt," he tells me. "I would never see them in the emergency department. So we always make this assumption that, you know, mental illness leads to suicidal thinking, leads to suicide, like it's these concentric circles." In fact there may be a Venn diagram, with some expressing distress and getting help, and others acting on impulse without ever showing outward signs.

It might take years for us to understand all the mental health impacts of 2020. Whatever protections adults—and apparently, some white people—experienced did not extend to children, teenagers, and young people of color. Or perhaps the protection they did experience was not strong enough to shelter them from the headwinds they were staring down at the same time.

FINDING HOPE IN THE WORST-CASE SCENARIOS

I was not expecting to find a deep well of hope and optimism when talking to people who deal with death every day. But that's exactly what happened when I started contacting children's bereavement centers around the country.

Grief is not a mental disorder. It's a near-universal human experience—a stage in the cycle of love. But mental health support can be helpful in the process of mourning. And childhood bereavement, in particular, is classified as an adverse childhood experience, which raises lifelong risks to health. Tallying the impact of the pandemic on children's psyches includes this kind of loss.

A CDC epidemiologist estimated that COVID itself bereaved at least 175,000 children in the United States from April 2020 to the fall of 2021. It took away a parent or grandparent who took care of them. Two-thirds of these children were Black, Latinx, or Native American. Partly that was because people of color tended to die from COVID at younger ages. In general, from all causes, Black and Latinx children are much more likely than white children to lose someone important to them in an untimely way.

Globally, the figure of children losing caregivers to COVID was estimated at 1.5 million, a mass orphaning comparable to that produced by the AIDS crisis at its height. And also consider the children who lost their dear ones to other causes during lockdowns who weren't able to call on the normal rituals of grief or places of social support.

In Chapter 5, you met the Alfaros, a Mexican American family in San Antonio, Texas. In the years before the pandemic, the children shared a bedroom with their papi. They weren't able to visit after he was hospitalized for COVID. When he died in July 2020, Crystal Alfaro had to call all over town to find a funeral home that would do an in-person service. And when she found one, the place was so busy they had to wait three more weeks. It was important to

Crystal to have the closure of a funeral, since she hadn't been able to be at her father's bedside when he was sick. Twelve-year-old Christian felt the same way. Fourteen-year-old Gisele was more hesitant but did decide to go to the funeral and said that she was glad that she did.

After the rosary service, some of their close family friends came back to the house for dinner. "It's an older couple, my in-laws' age," says Javi, the children's father. "And he was talking to us about when he lost his dad and he went through bereavement counseling. And he said it's nothing to be ashamed of—it's something that helped me."

Javi Alfaro says that their friends helped them overcome some cultural conditioning that might have stopped them from seeking professional help. "Being Hispanic, I think there's that strong, 'I don't need to go to the doctor. I don't need to talk to somebody'—and I've just got to realize that it's OK." Their family friend told them about the Children's Bereavement Center of South Texas.

A few dozen centers around the country specialize in grief counseling for children and their families. They are often free and funded by donations. The Children's Bereavement Center of South Texas is one of the largest and oldest, having been around for a quarter century. It is a catchment basin for the rivers of trauma, individual and collective, that well up in this part of the country. It serves migrant children who've recently crossed the border at its Rio Grande location. It opened a third location in 2017 after a mass shooting in a church in Sutherland Springs, Texas. "If you were able to be here and see our center, it's like a big warm home," Tami Logsdon, the program director, tells me. "In ordinary times you would smell dinner cooking with volunteers. We have pet therapy dogs." Of course for most of 2020 it went virtual.

The center provides both group and individual therapy for children as young as three years old, as well as for their caregivers. This part of Texas was so hard hit by COVID that the center started COVID-specific online support circles.

At the beginning the Alfaros were most concerned about Christian, their artistic, sensitive younger son. "He was crying, he was sad. He was really hurting and voicing that he was hurting," says his mom.

"I'm really open about everything, so as soon as my mom told me about the treatment center and that we could get help, I was really excited about it," Christian says. "I didn't know what it could lead me to. And I think without it, I wouldn't be where I'm at right now, and I wouldn't be as happy as I am. They really helped me get my way through grief."

He learned "that it's OK to cry, because before I feel like crying would be breaking down, and I learned that crying can let out your emotions because if you bottle them up, then it could maybe cause some mental issues. Crying is OK. It's not bad."

Over time, the parents came to realize that Gisele, who was more reluctant, was the one who really needed to open up.

Gisele says she learned that all her emotions were OK—if she was sad, or angry, or even happy. That she wasn't alone and she wasn't "weird" for feeling a certain way. And the circles made it safe for her to talk about what the therapist called "her person" and hold on to the good memories.

It was really important to the whole family to have other people to talk to who had experienced the losses of COVID directly, because they were surrounded by people who didn't take the disease seriously and didn't care to follow the rules or wear masks.

Gradually the whole family started to feel better. After a rough start to the remote school year in the fall of 2020, Gisele and Christian found their teachers to be supportive and understanding, and they were able to dig in and pull their grades up. Christian even got involved in drama club, creating remote newscasts with other students.

GRIEF COMES OUT OF THE SHADOWS

Bereavement counselors told me that they were experiencing a huge surge of interest and donations during the pandemic.

They saw the potential for the post-COVID world to become a more tender place.

"For those of us who are in the bereavement field, there is some hope, in that bereavement has come out of the shadows in many ways," Micki Burns, the chief clinical officer of Judi's House in Denver, Colorado, tells me. "So whereas before to talk about grief and loss and death, people would sometimes blow it off, you know, and say, 'Didn't that happen like a year ago? Aren't you over that already?'"

And now, "with the mass amount of death that we've seen, it has really created this place of empathy and understanding for families who were grieving before, and even more so for families who have had a loss in the past year or so."

Everyone lost something during this pandemic. It's one of the few events in human history to affect every living person on earth. We are all grieving in different ways. Holding that simple fact up to the light is an invitation to heal together.

"I have a bumper sticker that says, 'Connection is the cure,'" Melinda Macht Greenberg, the clinician in Massachusetts, tells me. "It's having that connection with other people that helps us get through tough times, whatever those problems are."

Connection is the cure. And vulnerability is strength. It's possible that our kids are already showing us the way forward here. There are researchers who believe that the upward trends in depression and suicide among youth, which started in the late 2000s, may be partly an improvement in diagnosis. Because of changes in the culture, like the waning of macho stereotypes, younger people are more apt to voice their needs and their feelings. Certain deaths, maybe, are no longer labeled accidents, because families aren't ashamed anymore to say what actually happened.

Jeannie tells me she suspected Rob thought it was "trendy" to have a therapist and talk about mental health problems. That comment made me think about Jeannie's history. Coming from multiple generations of mental illness and trauma, a teen mother herself, who became a present and self-aware mother to her own children, one who struggles with, seeks treatment for, and talks openly about trauma, depression, and anxiety. She had a young son who spoke up to a friend when he was in pain. That friend knew that they could and should go to a school counselor for help. And Rob and his mother accepted the help. That is indeed a trend—a positive trend.

MENTAL HEALTH IS PUBLIC HEALTH

A policy organization called Child Trends put out a publication in early 2021 proposing a new national agenda for children's mental health, post-pandemic.

Open up from a narrow focus on treatment and crisis response. Go upstream, to prevention for entire communities.

Open up from individual children alone to offering help to their families, as the Children's Bereavement Center of South Texas does.

Open up from mental health needs alone to the interrelation between mental and physical health and basic needs like housing. Break down silos between agencies and coordinate services, as Nick Chandler is doing at Buena Vista Horace Mann.

Educate everyone. Give people a basic vocabulary for talking about mental and emotional pain, how it shows up, and how to respond. Make a point of offering help to everyone, the ones who are up front about their distress like Christian and the ones who bottle it up like his big sister, Gisele.

Burns says that during the pandemic, Judi's House created a bereavement education program for entire schools. "We talk about, what is grief, and what is it like to experience grief, what is our reaction, and how can you be a support to a friend who is grieving? How do you know when your friend might need more help than what you can provide and you need to reach out to an adult?"

That way, when a second grader loses a parent, they aren't coming back to school with classmates who avert their eyes. This training also gives teachers the tools they need to support grieving students, which most say they aren't prepared to do. "To be like, OK, I can open up these conversations in my classroom and we can support kids who are grieving in the classroom. It doesn't have to be all on the counselor. It can be something that we do together as a community. We see it as a universal prevention program. Let's help to create a very sensitive community."

HEALING BY LISTENING

We can't presume to define the experience of any young person. It is up to them to say what a loss means to them, or to say how they feel about anything, for that matter. And how they feel in the moment likely will change over time and in unpredictable ways.

Ebony, the sixteen-year-old in New Orleans, tells me the same thing. "I would want adults to know that it pays to be empathetic. Because I think that sometimes adults...they have these stereotypes. I think that it pays to listen to what we have to say, especially if it involves our health."

Joseph Kelly, the director of programs at Peter's Place in Delaware County, Pennsylvania, says listening is key to his practice. He tells me about an approach that he takes to grief counseling, from author and educator Alan Wolfelt. It's known as "companioning." "We are not the experts on your grief. You are. And we seek to understand that through inquiry and through listening. The goal of companioning isn't about finding your way out. It's about honoring the journey as you walk it."

This is as true for bereavement as it is for general mental health struggles and other obstacles that young people faced during the pandemic. We adults may regret what children were put through. We may be angry about how leaders or institutions failed them. We may feel guilty or overwhelmed by sadness. But we owe them the respect of allowing them to claim the meaning of their own experience. Even if it hurts us to see them hurting, we can't rush them out of the process of coming to terms with what happened, let alone moving beyond it.

In our brief conversations, Ebony impressed me with her sense of purpose and independence. It seemed to me that she wasn't trying to get rid of her anxious nature—instead, she was channeling it, letting it power her forward. "I'm a very strong individual. I'm the type of person to push past my emotions. The hospital was the very last straw, because usually I'm very good at focusing on me and what I need to know and the bigger picture. That's what keeps me going, is having that goal for myself."

WINTER 2020–2021

10   POLITICS

Shout out to all the parents making breakfast, turning on PBS Kids, singing songs, & keeping tiny people balanced and protected in the midst of all of this.

> —Joshua DuBois, @joshuadubois,
> November 4, 2020, 15.9K Likes

January 10, 2021, US seven-day average of cases: 254,877

I lived through it. You—unless you are reading this many years in the future, maybe for a school assignment—lived through it. But it was too much to take in all at once. Election. Insurrection. Vaccines. Storms. And looming behind all of it, death. From early December all the way through mid-February, Americans died of COVID, very often at a rate of one 9/11—three thousand souls—per day.

The nation's children witnessed all of this. We tried to sequester them from the luridly incomprehensible. We held fast to the brief moments of celebration and hope, sparkling in the darkness.

November 3, 2020, saw the highest voter turnout not only in numbers but in percentage of eligible voters since 1900. The winner, Joe Biden, ultimately received a record eighty-one million votes.

Five-year-old PJ had a grand time on Election Day. He was out at the polls with his whole family from seven in the morning, telling people to vote for his mom.

With DC public schools still remote, Patricia had used her time to get even more involved in her community. She was gunning for Advisory Neighborhood Commission, an unpaid, two-year term advising the city on matters affecting her Deanwood neighborhood. "I live here and I'm always low-key complaining. Why not be a part of the process of change?" she explains.

Patricia lost by just seventy-one votes to another, more seasoned, male local politico who had lost a bid for City Council and came back to reclaim his ANC seat. Patricia felt like sexism was part of the reason.

"I didn't expect for so many people to keep asking me about, like, where's my husband or where's my children," when she was out campaigning, she says. "It was just like, wow. So I can't be a leader? I can't be interested in politics? I kept feeling like I was being told to 'stay in your place.'"

Patricia quickly recovered her optimism. She frames the whole thing as a learning experience. "It's frustrating, but…that's OK. There's always next time. I am definitely running again. My goal is to one day sit on the [City] Council."

The presidential election was a different story. Patricia describes her mood about it as "somber." "I didn't even want to look at the results or what the Electoral College did. I remember my very first time I voted and I voted for Al Gore. And then I found out, like, Florida did Florida and he didn't win. So that's always been kind of in the back of my head—I hope this doesn't get Gored up."

November 4, 2020, shortly after 2:00 a.m.: Donald Trump gives a speech in which he falsely claims victory: "We were getting ready to win this election. Frankly, we did win this election. We did win this election. So our goal now is to ensure the integrity for the good of this nation."

What Julian, at seventeen, in Oklahoma, hated most about the pandemic was how everything seemed to come back to politics. He calls himself a centrist compared to his parents, who were committed Democrats. His girlfriend's family was mostly Republican. Some of his coworkers at Sonic were Trumpers. "Some are pro-mask for the sake of safety, and they're oftentimes called sheep, and the others are just called idiots. Everything's just become a very hot-button kind of issue. At work, almost every other hour, someone has to bring up a political issue and then it turns into a debate. Everyone just starts talking and talking and talking about it. I kind of get sick of it."

His brother, Rob, at fourteen, was caught up in the drama too. "One of my friends, she's very leftist. She cuts anyone out of her life that are Trump supporters."

After November 3, the arguments didn't end: at home, at Sonic, among Rob's friends over Xbox, or at school. If anything, the volume got turned up even more. One of Jeannie's cousins maintained on Facebook that the election was stolen. Jeannie felt more and more alienated from friends, family, coworkers, the parents of her students. It was a small town, hard for anyone to keep their opinions to themselves.

November 7, 2020: As votes are being counted, there are dueling rallies in Philadelphia and elsewhere between Democratic activists chanting "Count Every Vote" and Republican activists chanting "Stop the Steal." Rudy Giuliani, the president's lawyer, holds a press conference outside a landscaping company located on the same block as a sex shop and across the street from a crematorium. He repeats the president's baseless allegations of election fraud. "Networks don't get to decide elections, courts do," he says.

It felt to Julian like he was seeing the bad side of everyone. He was angry all the time and tired of being angry, and being angry made him even more tired. He had a showdown with Jeannie just before the election. He told her he might have voted for Trump if he had been old enough. Jeannie had always prided herself on being the kind of parent who lets their kids think for themselves. But she couldn't take Trump for an answer. They debated, hotly, and he finally quieted her down with "Am I not allowed to have my own opinion in this house?"

Jeannie called him rebellious. They'd been fighting anyway over grades and over whether Julian was going to go to college at all or move out and rent his own apartment in Tulsa. Jeannie didn't see that happening on a fast-food wage. She didn't think Julian understood anything about the real world.

November 7, 2020: Pennsylvania and the nation are called for Joe Biden. Kamala Harris becomes the first woman, the first Black person, and the first person of South Asian descent to be elected vice president. People pour into the streets in celebration in New York, Los Angeles, Philadelphia, Atlanta, Washington, DC, and other Democratic-leaning cities around the country.

It was a straight line in Patricia's head from presidential politics to racial inequality, and to the need for more opportunities in her neighborhood.

> Why can't we do things the right way? Why isn't the Constitution a living, breathing document? Why aren't you holding everyone accountable to it? Why is there always two sets of laws and two types of justice? For four hundred years we've been here, we've been working, busting our ass, doing all this....I've met so many small business owners, so many entrepreneurs in Deanwood. And I'm like, wow, we have all this talent just sitting here, just chilling, like, how do you cultivate that talent?

November 9, 2020: Pfizer and BioNTech announce a COVID vaccine candidate has achieved a spectacular 90 percent efficacy against infection in phase 3 trials. The FDA had previously said that anything over 50 percent would receive approval.

COVID cases are rocketing upward for the worst phase of the pandemic yet seen in the United States. On Election Day, 92,416 cases are reported. Five days later, on November 8: 130,449 new cases. Schools that managed to open start going remote again around the country, and many will not open for several weeks into January.

At least the holidays brought a break. Jeannie doesn't like Thanksgiving because it reminds her how dysfunctional her family is. Usually the only family they see are her grandparents, and they only stay for an hour. This year she was going to drop off a plate at their place.

Otherwise, it would be basically the same as any other time: just her and the kids. "I feel bad for everybody else who's having to make all these changes and sacrifices. But for me, it's not any different."

Then she got inspired. "I love Halloween so much, and I do not love Thanksgiving because of the whole family thing. Halloween is fun. Thanksgiving is not. Our Halloween was so terrible, we didn't get one, so I tried to do something different; I said, let's celebrate Halloween during Thanksgiving week."

They had their Christmas tree up and decorated early, plus a Halloween tree right next to it with spooky decorations. They listened to scary stories and music. They had a life-sized skeleton, cobwebs on the piano, and a piñata shaped like the coronavirus. "It's really kind of bananas."

The kids chose the menu: turkey, green bean casserole, dressing. Ruby helped make the pies: tomato, Shoney's strawberry Jell-O, pumpkin, pecan, and cherry.

Heather, in St. Louis, couldn't make Thanksgiving dinner because she didn't have a working refrigerator. "We didn't get a chance to enjoy our Christmas or Thanksgiving. I didn't get to do the type of cooking my family prides itself on." They had to put their milk and cheese out on the back step and hope it stayed cold enough.

November 30, 2020: Results are in for the Moderna vaccine. Efficacy against COVID-19 is an astonishing 94.1 percent.

On Thursday, December 2, Oklahoma governor Kevin Stitt declared a "day of prayer and fasting" for those affected by the pandemic. It made Jeannie feel "catty." She baited her ultraconservative coworkers, saying, "Oh, tomorrow's going to be wonderful, guys, because everybody in Oklahoma is fasting and praying and so our cases are going to go down." And she staged her own little protest too. "As soon as I got up, I got a big bowl of cereal. That was my rebellion. And then I prayed for [Stitt] to grow some brain cells."

The day of prayer and fasting didn't work. In fact at one point in December, Jeannie checked the *New York Times* and saw her county was something like number 17 in the nation for new cases.

Not surprisingly for an English teacher, Jeannie is a big reader. She's been working her way through a list she printed off the internet called "1000 Books to Read Before You Die." One of her favorites is *One Hundred Years of Solitude.* "I kind of like that surreal fiction where you're not quite sure what's real, what's not. Not total fantasy. That's too much."

But over the winter she felt like she was surrounded by magical thinking, and not in a good way.

There was the superintendent of Oklahoma schools, who had decided that COVID-positive students could be quarantined at school in a classroom together. And the local district leadership, which declared that after Christmas there would be no more distance learning, period, no matter what happened.

There were the people who sprayed Lysol around instead of wearing masks, who talked about taking ivermectin, who said of COVID, " 'I'll go when it's my time to go.' Well, you know, OK, that's fine. You can die. But what about the people that you spread it to?"

Jeannie traced this mentality back to Oklahoma's original white settlers.

"If you look at our history, we're called Sooners because, you know, they ran the land and claimed land early." In 1889 the federal government held a run on lands appropriated from Plains Indians and other tribes, handing out 160 acres apiece, first come, first served. Sooners were the people who jumped the starting gun to stake their claims. "So, like, we have a history of only looking out for number one...like from the very beginning."

Mid–December 2020: The United States reaches a grim milestone: 250,000 new cases a day.

Dara Kass, in New York City, was watching the case counts grow around the country. She felt exasperated, like people were giving up on even trying to contain the virus.

Among other worries, she knew she'd have to cut back on the plans for Hannah's bat mitzvah in December. This was a direct result of something Hannah often groused about—the MSNBC effect.

With Dara appearing regularly on TV as a public health advocate, and giving advice privately to the kids' schools, their synagogue, friends, acquaintances, and strangers, she knew her family's own COVID choices were under a microscope.

As a doctor, she could have asked a large group of friends and family to quarantine and take multiple tests before gathering for the bat mitzvah. But as a matter of principle, "I did not want to test to have a party. Even if I could figure out a way for it to be truly safe, like they were doing in the NBA or whatever, it wasn't reproducible for the real world. That was not the right answer for lots of people. And I felt like a lot of the decisions I made needed to be because people were watching." This bothered Hannah, because it felt like her mom sometimes chose appearances over what would have made her, and the family, happiest.

They scaled back to just extended family at the synagogue for the service, followed by a lunch with each nuclear family seated at their own table. The kids' party, which in a regular year might have resembled a mini-prom, was a dinner for eight of Hannah's friends at a high-end sushi restaurant in Tribeca. There was a last-minute swerve when the restaurant declared the weather would make outdoor seating impossible. Ultimately, they were seated in semiprivacy behind a curtain. The girls still made the most of it and got dressed to the nines. Hannah had her hair blown out and wore a sparkly tiara.

"I thought it was actually good, but it definitely was not what I imagined it to be," Hannah equivocated. "Although it was still the best it could possibly be, it was kind of annoying, I guess, because I pictured everybody being together, and I have, like, this big party and all the people in the temple, like the temple is filled. But that's not how it was. It was obviously different, like the times that we're in, but it was the best it could have possibly been, like, I had the people who I really cared about around me."

Dara was most relieved when it was all over. It felt like they got it done just in time. As cases mounted, she felt the need to scale back the family's schedule even more. Playdates would only be allowed with the kids they were in school with. Hannah could meet up and go for walks if it wasn't too cold.

The family spent the holidays at home, just the four of them, with the presents bought and wrapped by Dad.

Their family tradition is to alternate giving and getting for the eight nights of Hanukkah. On "give" nights each kid presents a charity of choice, and they pick one for the family to donate to.

On the first night, December 10, they donated to Sammy's choice, a soup kitchen and women's shelter near their home in Brooklyn.

Dara seethed watching people in their social circle head off for winter beach getaways as ICU beds filled up once again. She posted on Facebook:

> You may be testing every single day, flying on a private plane or driving for 36 hours straight, but your random Facebook friends don't know anything about your plan. They just know you are on vacation. It also makes it really hard for us who are telling our kids that travel isn't safe this year to not look like overly cautious bad guys. Basically, if you are going on vacation this December, despite the draw of Facebook and Instagram, can you please just keep it to yourself.

A kid in Sammy's basement class had tested positive. But his symptoms were mild, and no one else in the room got it. The whole experience, while frightening, ultimately strengthened Dara's confidence that spread in schools could be effectively mitigated.

She thought schools needed to update their guidance; they were sending far too many kids home to quarantine for each case. In her opinion it was unnecessary, frustrating, and harmful.

> We're basically preventing the spread of the virus, but not keeping operation viability. We needed the Department of Education and the Department of Health and Human Services to get together with the CDC and have really, really important guidelines for the state of

our children that take into account spread in schools, the educational needs of our kids, risk mitigation, investment testing, investment in PPE—I mean, this should have just been done so differently.

December 11, 2020: The FDA issues an emergency authorization for the Pfizer vaccine.

December 14, 2020: Sandra Lindsay, a Black critical-care nurse at Long Island Jewish Medical Center, becomes the first American to receive a COVID vaccine outside of a clinical trial.

December 18, 2020: The FDA issues an emergency authorization for the Moderna vaccine.

Jeannie's neighbor, one of her only friends, had "gone over to the dark side" with conspiracy theories. Jeannie could laugh along when she was talking about aliens coming to visit Earth during the "star of Bethlehem." That was the rare planetary alignment of Jupiter and Saturn that blazed in the night sky, just to the left of the crescent moon, on the winter solstice of 2020. It gave the world a tiny little reprieve from talking about COVID, stolen elections, or the dawn of American fascism; but it could definitely be read as an omen, if you were into that sort of thing.

Jeannie's laughter got a little more nervous when the neighbor started sending her QAnon memes on TikTok and telling her Tom Hanks was a child molester who left his wife for a porn star. And she was pretty upset when the neighbor told her the vaccine was a Trojan horse, that "Bill Gates is going to implant the mark of the beast into us." Jeannie worried that lots of her community would feel the same way.

"People are worried about there being a shortage for the vaccine, you know, but we'll have a surplus here, really. I don't know of anybody who's willing to get the vaccine," she told me in January. Trump supporters were onto the Bill Gates stuff, and the Trump haters were skeptical because Operation Warp Speed was his project. "We've been taught or been told not to trust the government for four years."

A VIGIL FOR CARMELO DUNCAN

Late in the evening of December 2, a fifteen-month-old boy was fatally shot in Southeast Washington, DC, while strapped into a car seat in the back of a car driven by his father. News reports suggested it was a targeted attack, with the car struck several times. Patricia, of course, thought of her little boy Patrick, almost the same age. And she had an even closer connection—she had been a summer camp counselor for the baby's eight-year-old brother, who was in the car next to him and survived.

She wanted to go to the memorial and balloon release for the little boy. Really, she felt like she needed to go. It was a chance to mark not only this but a string of other recent violence and losses.

The death of this cherub-cheeked toddler was part of a surge in violent killings in DC and around the nation in 2020. The nation's homicide rate was up by one-quarter in 2020, a massive increase, taking it back to levels last seen in the late 1990s. Nationwide, 46 percent of victims were Black, although they make up just 13.4 percent of the US population.

Patricia had her own personal tally. There was a colleague who had died of cancer in March. Shantel Hill, a twenty-eight-year-old former parent at her school, was shot and killed, and yet another little child she knew, a two-year-old girl, was stabbed in a terrifying random attack, both in May.

"I just wanted to be there with people. Other than this, I'm not really hanging out or being around people."

Her husband, Pete, was completely against it. He was worried for her safety twice over: from COVID cases rising and from people who might be drawn to the gathering to continue the cycle of violence. He lost his temper.

The pandemic stress was getting to their marriage. In general Patricia felt really grateful for Pete. For his part, he tells me, "She's an amazing woman. I've learned a lot from her."

They had gotten together after college, but they knew each other from growing up in the Seventh-Day Adventist community in Los

Angeles. Pete had actually followed a different girl out east. When he started paying attention to Patricia, sweet and handsome as he was, she couldn't believe he was serious. "I thought I'd always be a round-the-way girl," she says, someone to hook up with, not to stick with. They struggled. "I got hurt at Peapod [a grocery delivery service] when one of the boxes flew off the conveyor belt and hit me. I couldn't work. We lived together in my car for a while until it got towed 'cause I took a car title loan out on it."

But they were here, together, all these years later.

They went to their pastor for counseling. They talked everything through and got to a better place. Pete wanted her to be more direct and up front with him about her plans, and she promised to do that.

Patricia went to the vigil and put some of it on Facebook Live. She talked to a Ward 8 City Council member and yet another woman who'd lost a child to violence. It was heavy. "I wouldn't want that to be me. And I wouldn't wish that on anyone else."

The month was an avalanche of stressors, big and petty. Patrick's daycare had several staff test positive and had to close for a long quarantine. PJ's asthma flared up when the winter weather set in, and he had to skip wrestling, which was an important outlet for his energy.

Then there was their next-door neighbor in the duplex. He was breeding puppies. One night in mid-December, fleas got through the pipes somehow and bit the boys up in their beds, worrying at them so badly that no one got much sleep. Patricia was up at the crack of dawn—Pete left for work at five thirty, so she was all alone. She put the boys in the bathtub, with bubbles and Alexa playing music to entertain them, while she stripped the beds, opened the windows, and tried to beat back the infestation. At one point she looked in the mirror—she was coughing, her face was bright red. She stuck her head under the faucet to try to snap out of it.

Patricia always knew how to look for silver linings. Some of the sports games she refereed had come back in person, and she was also making money doing deliveries for DoorDash and for some local businesses. Even before the second stimulus checks came, they had caught up on their car note and some other bills. She was able to budget and get presents under the Christmas tree. PJ, at five, still believed in Santa Claus. He was getting some new wrestling shoes, a flannel shirt for the cold weather, and a remote-controlled helicopter.

December 29, 2020: The second set of economic stimulus payments start going out. It's been eight long months since families last saw cash relief from the federal government.

Finally, Heather got a new fridge a few days before Christmas, but around the same time, she also got a letter from her landlord. It said they weren't going to renew her lease. As far as Heather could understand, they were out because her twelve-year-old son Shadrack had taken a neighbor's PlayStation. He told his mom that it was a present from his grandma. Heather made him give it back and even offered the neighbor some money, too, but the landlord didn't seem to care. Unless she could go to the right office, speak with the right supervisor, she feared losing her housing yet again.

Heather visited enough clothing and toy drives to make a good Christmas for the kids. She posted a picture on Facebook of her fifteen-year-old daughter holding her two-year-old daughter. The living room was cleaned up; there was a tree with lavender and silver ornaments, and stacks of presents: a kitchen play set, a scooter.

When Heather got her second stimulus check in December, she spent part of it on food for the folks living in a large tent encampment outside a vacant warehouse downtown. "We've been going down every once in a while, every time we can. We try to bring food for about twenty-five people."

She took Shadrack there with her in January, when the people living in the encampment got an eviction notice. "I want him to be on the front line with me, you know, let him know how important it is to make sure everyone has a safe, secure home." Heather was still trying to start her own business or nonprofit helping the homeless. It was hard to figure out the details; she was worried that her application for a business license would mess up her unemployment checks.

January 5, 2021: Jon Ossoff and Raphael Warnock win their runoff elections in Georgia, giving Democrats a fifty-vote majority in the Senate.

January 6, 2021: Trump addresses a rally of his supporters just south of the White House, and says, "If you don't fight like hell, you're not going to have a country anymore."

On the afternoon of January 6, Jeannie got a text from her oldest son, in Tulsa, telling her to turn on the news. It was a gymnastics day, so she and Ruby listened to the reports in the car. Jeannie remembers tearing up at several points, in shock and horror.

The attack on the US Capitol was the most documented political atrocity in American history. The Zapruder film of John F. Kennedy's assassination in 1963 was just twenty-six seconds long; this was livestreamed on social media, in real time, for hours, by thousands of participants and broadcast by journalists who were themselves trapped inside the building. The mob's stated intention was to disrupt the final certification of election results. Some Trump supporters were dressed in furs and face paint. Others were heavily armed. They brandished QAnon, Nazi, and Confederate flags. Rioters assaulted both reporters and police officers. One rioter was shot dead by Capitol police. The business of Congress was interrupted as lawmakers fled and hid. The election results were not certified until the wee hours of the morning.

"Why are they doing this?" Ruby wanted to know. The Black Lives Matter protests had made sense to her, but this kind of destructiveness she couldn't fathom. Jeannie regretted that her daughter had to see her so upset, with no answers to give.

Other people in her community did have answers. Jeannie's ex-husband's coworkers at the feed mill said that the Democrats had dropped off the protesters, that they were impostors there to make Trump look bad; and in the same breath they'd say, if Black Lives Matter protests were all fine, then the insurrectionists were fine, too, just expressing their First Amendment rights.

Jeannie heard many of the same opinions from her students, parroting what they'd heard at home. She knew she'd get complaints from parents if she pushed back too much; she had to pick her battles, deciding when to present them with facts, when to pretend to be deaf, and when to shut the conversation down.

If Jeannie had been teaching in person on Inauguration Day, she knew she wouldn't have risked watching it with her class. Too many of their parents thought Trump should still be president.

She watched it at home with a different sort of trepidation. "I turned it on and we were watching it and I kept thinking, if something horrible happens, my girls are going to see it firsthand. Is this what I want? And I thought, yes, I need to watch it. It was a risk."

MAGA COMES TO GOOD HOPE ROAD

The exact moment stuck in her head: at 2:38 p.m. on January 6, Patricia got an automated text message from the mayor announcing a curfew. She checked social media and realized that some of the protesters were perilously close to Patrick's daycare, on Good Hope Road, so she left immediately to go pick up her kids. "Running around, you know, you can see the anxiety in people's faces. They're rushing their kids out the door, grabbing jackets—we don't know what's coming, but we know that they're basically cool with just walking up to people—like, Tamir Rice was shot for playing with a toy gun, so." A twelve-year-old Black boy murdered by police in 2014 was on her mind as she worried what might happen to her own sons in the path of heavily armed MAGA protesters in paramilitary gear.

Patricia had expected something to go down, but she was shocked to see the rioters actually breach the Capitol. Why did the police, who brought maximum force to peaceful Black Lives Matter protests the previous summer, suddenly stand down? "If they were Black, they never would have made it in. I've seen ushers do a better job in churches. I honestly believe somebody was in on it. Somebody just told them something."

She was transfixed by the video that circulated on social media of Eugene Goodman, a Black Capitol Hill police officer, singlehand-edly fighting off a mob. "He's backing up all the time. You can see on his face he's like, oh shit. I can't fire my gun. It may ricochet. It may blow my eardrum out from the sound. You know, it's too many people. I'm outmanned. What can I do?"

On the one hand, she thought all this might somehow lead to a better conversation about police being trained in de-escalation tac-tics and about reducing gun violence. Now that it was white people yelling about their First Amendment right to protest, maybe people would listen.

On the other hand, the political forecast was bleak in her opinion. "The sad part is there's going to be a smarter racist young white man that's paying attention that's going to probably try to replace Trump."

January 13, 2021: The House of Representatives impeaches Donald Trump on a single count: "incitement of insurrection." He becomes the first president ever to be impeached for the second time. Ten House Republicans vote in favor.

January 20, 2021: Joe Biden is inaugurated without incident.

The winter dragged on. Heather's youngest son, the baby king and everyone's favorite, was walking. Then the pipes burst in the base-ment. They had to boil their drinking water for over a month. "Some-times I laugh to keep from crying."

February 15, 2021: Presidents' Day, a massive winter storm hits. Weather-wise, this winter will be the costliest on record, with severe storms leading to a power crisis in Texas and at least 235 deaths around the country.

St. Louis got eight inches of snow and Heather's heat failed. "It was bone cold in here. We could see ourselves talk in the kitchen. We barely could come out of our room. We couldn't bathe. We couldn't hardly do anything."

Heather had a small space heater in her room that flickered like a fireplace. She piled the kids on her bed and put on some of the '80s sitcoms she used to watch with her mom. "We still ended up having a peaceful time, but it was so, so cold in here."

What happened next, Heather tells me, is a story of "how good God is."

She decided to go out and look for another space heater. They were all sold out at the Family Dollar nearby. She caught the bus out to Walmart. Sold out. Lowe's. Sold out. Home Depot. Sold out. She caught a ride back home for ten dollars from some boys at the Kwik Trip.

The next day she decided to check back at the Family Dollar, because she needed a mop anyway. She was walking back across the street with her mop over her shoulder and someone in a truck slowed down trying to talk to her. At first she thought it was some guy trying to flirt. But it was a woman with her daughter, offering her a ride home. Heather explained her situation, and the lady brought her to a couple more places to look for a heater. When they couldn't find one, the lady remembered she had an old one in her own house. She went over and got it for Heather, so they didn't have to spend another night in the cold.

SPRING 2021 AND BEYOND

11   FUTURE

Under the vast glass-and-steel roof of the former Union Station in downtown St. Louis sprawls a family amusement center with an artificial lake, a rope course, an aquarium, and a two-hundred-foot Ferris wheel. I visited with Heather and seven of her children in June 2021. The older children carried the younger ones. The seventeen-year-old had a diaper or two shoved in the pocket of his jeans.

Outside it was sweltering. Two-year-old Shekitha got scared and started shrieking when we plunged into the darkness of the aquarium. Standing in line, Heather cradled her gently until she quieted. As we walked from tank to tank, voices dropped to murmurs. We gazed for a long time at the nurse sharks, our faces bathed in eerie blue light. In the activity area, Habersham and his sisters cut out and colored fish-shaped paper crowns. Shadrack, at thirteen, was not too old to be amazed by petting the stingrays.

Heather had dressed everyone up for the occasion, the little girls in matching brand-new, tropical-print dresses. She had on a lemon-yellow shirtdress and strappy sandals. She was taking the whole family to be baptized the next day. Neither she nor her teens were vaccinated, though. She said she didn't believe in vaccines, in general. As a housing-insecure Black mother below the poverty line, she belonged to several of the demographic groups least likely to be vaccinated for COVID in the first half of 2021. Missouri was also lagging behind other states in its vaccination rate.

We stopped for a snack, sitting on the balcony so we could watch a fire display spurting over the lake. Habersham passed up the soda because his football coach forbade it. His oldest brother showed me his TikTok, which featured funny memes about working at Chipotle. The baby wandered back inside through double doors; another family returned him before any of us noticed he was gone.

SHOTS AND CHECKS

In the spring of 2021, patches of blue sky and sunshine were peeking through the clouds that had hovered over the world for the past twelve months. The new president's agenda was summarized in three words: "shots and checks." The vaccine rollout brought high hopes, as did Biden's American Rescue Package, which passed at almost exactly the one-year mark of the pandemic, March 11, 2021. No Republicans voted for the bill.

This was a Denali of federal spending—a mountain even higher than the New Deal. It had some crucial provisions for children and families. Like a third round of stimulus checks, $1,400 per family, which rolled out as tax returns were processed.

In a desperate hour, the federal government had turned its pockets inside out. And for once, "trickle-down economics" became more like a refreshing waterfall. Between direct stimulus, extra unemployment benefits, and more food stamp money offered under both Trump and Biden, the Urban Institute calculated that pandemic aid would drive down US poverty in 2021 to the lowest level on record.

Children are the age group most likely to be living in poverty, and correspondingly, the poverty rate among children fell the most of any group: from 15 percent in 2018 to 5 percent in 2021. This meant that the families of children who were going hungry in April and May 2020 were more flush than they'd ever been the following year, even though millions of jobs had disappeared. Eviction moratoriums were also instrumental in keeping families in their homes.

All of this was temporary.

CUTTING CHILD POVERTY IN HALF

Biden's first big spending package introduced a new cash benefit. If made permanent—a big if—it was calculated to cut child poverty by more than half.

This would amount to a sort of Social Security but for children. Like Social Security, this money was nearly universal. It was designed to reach 94 percent of American children. It didn't carry the shame or stigma of welfare benefits. It was judgment-free and automatic.

It didn't require certifying and recertifying yourself as needy or worthy, performing gratitude to a neighbor or a pastor, pleasing a bureaucrat in some office, or proving anything at all about your love life. It would arrive automatically to everyone who filed a tax return (which could prove to be a big asterisk, especially for people who work in the informal economy). The money would be mailed out in monthly checks, $250 per child over age six and $300 per child under age six, beginning in July 2021.

In the past decade, randomized controlled trials have tested the effects of direct cash assistance, sometimes called universal basic income programs. These studies show that when people get reliable income, it tends to make their lives better. They spend more than before on fresh fruit and vegetables and less on alcohol and cigarettes. They save and invest in things like education so that they can earn more in the future. They work more, not less. It's even been shown that when you tell people the money is for children, they go ahead and spend more of it on their children.

In 2021, the payments reached sixty-one million children and reduced child poverty by about 30 percent. Then they expired.

SCHOOLS IN RECOVERY

By the fall of 2021, all the evidence we had—standardized test scores, information from learning software programs, attendance data, student grades, graduation rates, opinion polls of parents and teachers—supported the idea that children nationwide had learned less than they normally would have during the pandemic pause. They missed more school hours. They failed more courses. The students who were already behind lost the most. Students who stayed remote the longest, on average, learned the least.

There were also data voids. We knew little about what students had learned in social studies or science, for example. We didn't have good measures of social and emotional development either. The country had skipped what are usually mandated state math and reading tests in the spring of 2020. The Biden administration insisted children be tested in the spring of 2021. But the students we were the most worried about, those disengaged from school and attending sporadically if at all, were probably missing from the testing rolls, making the results less reliable.

The American Rescue Package shoveled $130 billion to K–12 schools for COVID recovery, plus another $10 billion just for coronavirus testing in schools. This was on top of $70 billion allocated during Trump's term. Schools had three years to spend it all. Money was earmarked to go to students most in need. There was an additional fount of $350 billion directly to states, some of which would make its way to schools as well.

In contrast to his predecessor, President Biden's secretary of education had spent most of his career in public schools, in the small city of Meriden, Connecticut. Miguel Cardona was known as a nurturing teacher and later a consensus-building leader who pushed for school reopening in his state.

But Cardona didn't have a unifying or revolutionary grand vision for school recovery. With the money it was handing out, the federal government suggested hiring more teachers and school counselors, fixing ventilation systems, upgrading school buses. Some schools renovated their weight rooms and athletic fields.

The feds backed approaches to address student losses mostly through extra time: tutoring, longer school days and years, and summer school. There's an intuitive logic to this. In special education law, it is called "compensatory services": a school district can be ordered to provide extra hours of therapy and education if it can be shown that a child was denied appropriate services in the past. Many parents of students in special ed pushed for compensatory services post-pandemic.

But polls showed most parents had little appetite for extra time at school. After more than a year of unsatisfying remote and interrupted in-person instruction, they didn't believe that the answer was a higher dose of traditional school. They were more concerned about other forms of loss: children's loneliness, confusion, uncertainty, sadness. Teachers, for their part, were burned out. Staff shortages were becoming acute.

COULD WE REINVENT SCHOOL?

The moment presented a fragile opportunity for reinvention in education, a field that's always oscillating between conservatism and progressivism. Justin Reich at MIT interviewed teachers, students, and parents about how they envisioned schools responding post-pandemic. Very few said that they would concentrate on bringing up standardized test scores. "Rather than a 'return to normal' or the targeting of a narrowly-conceived 'learning loss,' the students and educators in our study emphasized themes of healing, community, and humanity as key learnings from the pandemic year and essential values to rebuilding schools," Reich and his colleagues report. They recommended that school communities provide more counseling, spend more time on social and emotional learning, and bring students together to commemorate what they'd been through: to make artwork, paint memorial murals, tell stories, perform poems, plant gardens. "Reflect on the pandemic year, celebrate resilience, grieve what has been lost, and imagine how the lessons learned from a tumultuous year can inform more equitable, resilient school systems for the future."

This is a compelling vision. But there was a real tension here.

On the one hand, time-based standards for learning are inherently arbitrary. And the social and emotional pain of the pandemic is real, though it may be hard to measure. Letting go of anxiety or urgency about "learning loss" might free educators and students to reconnect with the higher purpose of school and deal with each other as human beings.

On the other hand, free public education lasts only so many years. And as children grow up, other life concerns take priority over school, especially if they aren't confident in the basics and aren't making meaningful progress. A child who can't read well by third grade is likely to be frustrated and disengaged by middle school. A teenager who fails just one class in ninth grade is far more likely to drop out of high school, with lifelong consequences for earnings, health, and happiness.

Harris, the kindergarten teacher in San Francisco, knew that she had several children who were far behind where they should have been by the end of the year. "I have three kids that have hardly come. I mean, they don't know a thing. I don't know how I can send them to first grade. It hurts me." But she was loath to recommend they repeat kindergarten, because she didn't want them to be separated from their age cohort and feel unsuccessful or bad about themselves. "It's a very difficult decision," she said. She was worried about children not getting the interventions they need. "I'm thinking about, what does this look like fifteen years from now, ten years from now? And one of the things is, maybe somebody skates under the radar. Like you've got a kid who can't sit still, and it's May. You know that there's a lot of reasons for that. But, you know, if you could have spotted them in August or September, it would have been a little different."

The effects of the pandemic on student learning were grossly unequal. In response, students deemed to be behind would often get more of the same: more "diagnostic" standardized testing and more uninspired remedial worksheets or drills on the computer.

In Oakland, community activist Lakisha Young diagnosed a failure of will. Why can't public schools provide effective instruction at the right dose and pace for each student and also help them heal emotionally?

Her organization was part of a coalition suing the state for denying equal education to low-income students and students of color during California's longest-in-the-nation remote learning. At the first hearing in June 2021, she says, the state asked the court to drop the suit, citing the coming federal relief money. "Basically, 'We're about to get a ton of money. So everything's going to be fine,' right? And we're like, no. We want input on how that money is spent, and we're modeling what that could look like in Oakland."

Her group, the Oakland Reach, had formed a virtual hub starting in the summer of 2020 and continuing through the school year. Parents supported parents; teachers gave individualized attention. There was technology troubleshooting and mental health counseling, plus online art and karate classes. Reading scores grew and families felt more emotionally supported at the same time. "And we want that replicated across the state, across the country, because urban districts, knowing what to do with all of this money is going to be a real problem. It's actually an amazing time of reckoning. Because once we get to, like, five years from now and kids still are reading on the same grade level, people are going to have some explaining to do."

Young also knew many families of color who were uncertain about or opposed to returning to public schools at all. After spiking in the fall of 2020, homeschooling had settled at a still historically high rate of 8 percent of all families by May 2021. The growth was driven by Black, Hispanic, and Asian American families, many of whom still didn't feel it was safe to return.

"THE SCHOOL IS MORE LIKE A FAMILY"

Not every school or district failed the challenges of COVID and remote learning. Guilford County, a large district in North Carolina, posted its highest high school graduation rate ever in 2021—91.4 percent. Baltimore City Schools graduated one-fifth more high school students from its summer semester program in 2021, compared to 2019.

Researchers studied the positive outliers. They found some common threads.

The first and most important was strong relationships. Emmanuel, in Brooklyn, tells me about Liberation, his high school, where he heard directly from someone every day through the depths of lockdown: "The school is more like a family than staff and students. We interact with each other; we talk to each other every day."

The second was instructional designs that made it easier to teach students just what they needed to know. Like small-group and one-on-one sessions, flexibility in scheduling, combinations of individualized and group work. And at a higher level, telling students about the learning goals for the course, prompting them to reflect on and evaluate their own progress.

Having a computer on hand for each student and a software system already in place was a good sign but not a sufficient proxy for this kind of innovative school planning. After Katrina, some New Orleans schools similarly found success in addressing missed learning by keeping up the grade-level pace and filling in extra review for students who needed it, rather than having them plod along with remedial work.

Elements of choice in what they studied and a sense of higher purpose could also help keep students engaged and attached to school. Like Jesse Hagopian, the high school teacher in Seattle, who was able to adapt his lesson plans to directly speak in the moment to students' experiences with the Black Lives Matter protests in June 2020.

Or like Ebony at the alternative high school in New Orleans, the Net. After she struggled with remote learning and her mental health in the spring of 2020, she was able to do "credit recovery" to stay on track for graduation by retaking online courses at a faster pace. She also reconnected with the school community once they were back in person through a leadership and student voice committee. And she got involved at a community farm, one of many internship and job opportunities for students at the school.

Most intangibly, schools that succeeded during this time were simply high-functioning places. They had strong leaders, hope, trust.

All these strengths served students well before COVID. They would serve students well in the recovery and in the future disasters and disruptions that are surely to come.

Schools in the United States undeniably learned and grew from the pandemic, in ways that were both humane and innovative.

Teachers and parents now had each other's cell phone numbers. Kids now had computers and hotspots. Teachers learned more about what students were going through at home; parents knew more about what teachers were doing and gained more confidence to help. With less time, teachers were often forced to cut out deadwood to focus on the essentials. Justin Reich called this "Marie Kondo-ing the curriculum," after the Japanese decluttering expert. Teachers had reinvented their jobs in a matter of weeks, and what they learned would stick with them.

One far-reaching and momentous transition: most of the colleges in the country made it possible to apply without SAT or ACT scores. College admissions didn't magically become equitable by dropping these exams, but the pandemic might just be the end of the hundred-year tyranny of the number 2 pencil and measuring someone's worth or aptitude by a scaled score on a bell curve.

Even before the pandemic there was a chorus calling for a robust reconsideration of both what schools teach and how they teach it. That is not yet what was happening writ large in the fall of 2021, despite some bright spots. Instead, schools were yet again forced into crisis mode by a still-uncontrolled pandemic.

THE CARE AGENDA

The US birthrate has been dropping since the late 1950s. In a typical recent year it fell 2 percent. In 2020 it fell twice as fast, 4 percent. It was a demographic signature of despair, written into the historical record like a wildfire recorded in a tree ring. It's hard to think of a year in recent memory in which having a baby would have taken a bigger dose of optimism and faith.

That's true even though the child tax credit, essentially a family allowance, was one of the most child-friendly policies Americans had ever seen. The Rescue Plan for schools was the biggest infusion of cash into the public school system in a generation.

There was a synergy between these programs too. Less material hardship means more children coming to school ready to learn.

But these might have been just an appetizer. In late April 2021, Senator Elizabeth Warren's exhortation from the summer of 2020 that "childcare is infrastructure" was actually put into the words of a proposal, known first as the American Families Plan.

This plan, as originally written, would vault the United States from the back to the front of the pack among wealthy countries when it comes to public spending on children. It included universal public preschool for both three- and four-year-olds, with a fifteen-dollar-an-hour minimum wage for teachers. On top of that, childcare subsidies would go out in both directions: to middle-class and working-class families to make the fees affordable and to providers to support better wages and better training. And last but not least, the Families Plan included universal, national, paid family leave for the very first time.

It's hard to process how big this would have been. And honestly, I don't feel like Americans really tried. After a year in which every parent and every employer acutely felt the absence of childcare, we didn't have a public conversation commensurate with the size of the changes on the table. Advocates said their piece, sure, but there was no massive Moms March; #CareEconomy never trended on Twitter.

Maybe it was because the Families Plan was rolled up inside an even bigger total federal package that included crucial investments in climate, infrastructure, and more. Maybe because the coverage of that package was dominated by the horse trading over the votes of two senators flush with corporate donations who seemed determined to oppose their party's president at any cost.

Or maybe because the people—let's be honest, the women—who might have rallied around this bill were really goddamned tired. And Americans in general were feeling angry and beaten down, worried over threats to democracy and voting rights, viral variants and vaccine hesitancy, and the mundane yet intolerable conditions of everyday life in the Anthropocene.

Still, on some other timeline, this could have been the signature accomplishment of an entire presidency. The American Families Plan offered more than practical assistance or economic investment. It drafted a new social contract unlike anything this country has ever seen. It was a long-delayed fulfillment of the hopes raised by the model day nursery at the Chicago World's Fair in 1893 and dashed when shipyard childcare centers were shuttered after World War II. It was a policy that would recognize and reward the carers who were laid off during the pandemic or else asked to work in circumstances of unknown safety while others stayed home.

A country with a solid staircase of federally funded, broad, and broadly popular programs taking families from the newborn stage through kindergarten would be a country where families with children don't feel completely forgotten and dismissed. Where mothers don't have their backs against the wall as they try to calculate the short- and long-term tradeoffs between caregiving and working for wages. Where differences based on racial discrimination narrow. And where all little children in the critical months and years of life get the focused attention and care that their bodies, brains, and hearts need to thrive.

I hope to see it someday.

ROAD TRIP

With these possibilities still gleaming on the horizon, once I was fully vaccinated, I traveled to Washington, DC, San Francisco, St. Louis, and Oklahoma to meet my families in person for the first time.

I had been reporting through a computer screen for thirteen months straight. Now I was in people's homes, for hours and days.

I felt thin-skinned, easily overwhelmed by the sensory immersion. Several conversations happened through tears.

When I first started talking to families for my book, everything was frightening, enraging, and numinous. I couldn't have known what would become of any of us. I've stressed this entire book that it didn't have to be this way. It didn't have to be this hard. We could have done so much more to protect and to prioritize children throughout this pandemic. There are hurts and losses I believe children will carry with them for a lifetime.

But—AND—it's also true that most of us survived. And the children didn't just survive. They grew. That's what children do, if given the slightest chance.

WASHINGTON, DC

I visited Patricia and her family on a fresh spring day. Daffodils pushed up between cinder blocks in neat front yards. We met outside, at the sparkling new Deanwood Community Center. Patricia had helped bring an outdoor art installation here, sponsored by the Smithsonian. It featured heroic, bigger-than-life-size black-and-white photographs of Black male paragons: Ta-Nehisi Coates, Miles Davis, LeBron James. She had a proprietary air; more than one person asked her for directions. One of the campaign flyers from her run for neighborhood commissioner was still stuck to a nearby telephone pole.

PJ was coming from football practice. His uniform had a matching mask. In the first few months of lockdown, he was eating all the time because he was sad and lonely, his mother told me. He gained weight. Now he was healthy, strong, full of energy. Keeping him in shoes was a feat. Pete figured his son might be bigger than he is one day.

Patricia spoke to her older son with both authority and respect, a mother who was used to being listened to.

"Excuse me, use your normal voice, please, I don't want you yelling at me—PJ, can you say excuse me? Do you have something to add to the conversation?" Polite as could be, PJ asked for a second doughnut.

She tells me that she'd become a more tolerant and patient mother during the pandemic. "At first I was really angry. It was a lot...then I started thinking about, how can I make this fun for my kids and for me? We dug up the front yard, planted flowers, revamped the backyard. We focused more on our own stuff. My youngest came a long way this year. From lying on his tummy to walking and running."

And her marriage was stronger than ever. They'd been having heart-to-heart talks, "adulting" together, assembling their dreams and plans for the future, including starting a business that helped other local businesses find permits and contractors, called Simply Stamper LLC.

At the beginning of lockdown she feared being stuck at home like a 1950s housewife or, worse, a maid. Instead, between working, volunteering, running for office, working out with a personal trainer, and picking up side gigs for extra cash, Patricia stretched in many different directions during 2020. She reclaimed her time and used it to further her goals for herself, her family, and her community.

Little Patrick reached for my hand as he ambled along. He had been back doing his therapy in person for a few months and seemed to be coming along well, hefting a fallen tree branch three times his size. He still had progress to make with his speech and with potty training.

Patricia wasn't thrilled about it, but she got her vaccine. She would leave the public schools for a position at a charter school. She was pulling PJ out of public school for the fall as well, and letting Theresa Garza keep educating him at her daycare. "I don't trust DCPS [DC Public Schools]," she said simply.

SAN FRANCISCO

When I got to their house, Jonah and Khamla were helping Maya in the garden as a Mother's Day present. The sky was blazing blue and the city fragrant with roses, hibiscus, and jacaranda. Maya was digging out succulents to bring to her new garden. The family was moving to the East Bay.

In late July, Maya and Robert got married in their living room.
They had been engaged for a couple of years before the pandemic.
It was small but sweet: the kids; Robert's parents; his sister and her
family; Thea's brother; her dad, who was so sunk in dementia that he
wouldn't remember the ceremony; and her mom, who was feeling
better for the moment.

The family celebrated in Hawaii—Khamla too. And then, all of a
sudden, a year after he joined the family, it was time for Khamla to go
home. His mother had found an apartment and not one but several
jobs and was eligible for "reunification," in the parlance of the family
welfare system.

The whole thing was painfully abrupt for Maya and Robert. In
the lead-up, Khamla was so nervous he was having panic attacks. But
once he and his mother were settled, together, in their new home,
something amazing happened. He invited Jonah for a sleepover.

OKLAHOMA

Jeannie's house was as cheerful and organized as a Pinterest board.
The living room was minimalist yet rustic, with a fireplace, white
walls, and a sisal rug. On the sideboard were bowls of quartz crys-
tals that the family gathers every summer on a hike to a beloved
mountaintop.

Ruby introduced me to the frogs, the cats, the dog, and the turtle,
Matilda. She prepared me a deconstructed strawberry pie, with sticks
of piecrust that you dip first into strawberry compote and then into
whipped cream. She also knit me a hat during my visit.

The "babies" seemed to have their own private language, like twins
sometimes do. They smiled to themselves, cuddling their mother on
the couch.

Rob was in fine spirits. He joked about a meme involving the pop
star Lizzo and gave his mother a hard time. He had been vaccinated,
so he could see his friends much more easily. In particular, there was
a certain girl who was really smart and funny, who wore elaborate

TikTok makeup, and whose hair was half black and half bleached blonde. She happened to be dating his best friend.

We drove to Sonic, where Julian was working.

"Hello, welcome to Sonic, may I take your order?"

"Julian, it's Mom. Come out and say hi."

"May I please take your order, ma'am?"

It was windy at the picnic table. An elementary school classmate of Jeannie's brought out our tater tots, cherry limeade, and freezes. Julian never showed.

He had had a tough few months. He and his girlfriend broke up right after prom. Julian's story was that she dumped him because of his temper. Jeannie didn't like the sound of that but also hoped the experience would teach him about how to treat women before he got much older.

He went back and forth about college all year. Finally he applied and was accepted to the Oklahoma State University Institute of Technology. But there was a problem. During the many months when school seemed pointless, Julian's GPA had declined to the point where he lost access to the Oklahoma's Promise scholarship program, which would have given him a free ride to public college in the state.

> He said he decided he was going to go to Oklahoma State University. And he had a Cherokee Nation scholarship. And so I kind of sat him down and I said, look, Julian, this is $2,400 a semester. You're getting $400 a semester.
>
> He was proud of his scholarship. But I did the math and I showed him how much he's going to go into debt. And I said, you probably should not do this. You should try junior college because you've already, like, shown us that you are not motivated. And until you are, you don't need to amass that debt.

She was serving up tough love, but inside Jeannie was distraught. Her oldest son had opted for the military over college and was still struggling financially and in other ways. Julian, her firstborn with her ex, George, was handsome, talented on the guitar, smart, and hardworking. She couldn't stand to see him throw away his future. But she didn't have the money to finance a pipe dream either.

He ended up moving out of the house and getting a full-time job in a factory. He told his mother he would sign up for junior college classes, but she didn't think he was putting much energy into it.

Julian had company. Undergraduate enrollment in the United States, which had dropped in fall 2020 by 4.3 percent, fell by another 3.5 percent in 2021. The young people whose higher education dreams are deferred by the pandemic, will, if history is a guide, go on to earn less money and have lives that are harder in other ways.

RACE AND HISTORY IN TAHLEQUAH

Jeannie and I drove to the capital of Cherokee Nation to get pizza and talk. Talequah is quaint, even a little hip. It's a college town; Northeastern State University was founded in 1851 as the Cherokee Female Seminary. The Cherokee National History Museum opened in 2019 in the old Capitol building, next to the Cherokee Nation's own courthouse. There's a historical timeline of the nation inlaid into the sidewalk. The street signs are in both Cherokee and English.

Our visit was right around the centennial of the Tulsa Race Massacre, when a white mob destroyed a prosperous Black neighborhood and killed as many as three hundred people.

Once relegated to a historical footnote, the event was being commemorated almost as though it were breaking news. Astonishingly, three survivors were there to testify to what had happened and call for reparations: Viola Fletcher, 107; her younger brother Hughes Van Ellis, 100; and Lessie Benningfield Randle, 106.

History is not simple. Part of the wealth that built Black Wall Street, the district that was the target of the Tulsa Race Massacre, originated in federal land allotments granted to freedmen who lived on Cherokee lands. One fact inscribed in the sidewalks of Tahlequah is that some of those freedmen were brought to the reservation lands in the first place as slaves by Native Americans who sided with the Confederacy.

Jeannie had a different kind of history on her mind and a different kind of wrong. She was plagued by the thought that she had left Julian and his brother essentially on their own to cope all year, as she focused on the more immediate needs of her younger children, not to mention her own mental health. Was it all because of the pandemic? Was it her divorce, her generational history of dysfunction? Could things have gone any differently, or better, if she'd just had more time or more help?

BROOKLYN AND SCARSDALE

Dara Kass's three kids were thrilled to be headed to camp for the summer, and she was even more thrilled to see them go. Testing, quarantining, and of course vaccines made it safe, in her judgment, even for Sammy. He would peel away from the video games, hang with his cousins, get some sunshine.

Hannah saw the chance to make up for some of the fun that had been lost in this strange year. She was saying goodbye to some people and going to a new school. Eighth grade hadn't been anything like she once pictured.

The family was moving to the suburbs. Dara wanted all three children in the same school system for the fall, with the same quarantine and testing rules. She changed her hospital shifts to the weekends so she could spend less time commuting and have more time for policy and public-facing work.

Dara also got on an airplane with Michael once they were fully vaccinated, and headed for a resort in Puerto Rico. Her first real vacation since December 2019. She couldn't believe how free she felt— so free that she actually got up from the beach chair once to head inside and forgot her mask for a minute. She didn't post any beach selfies to Facebook.

And she put in twelve-hour shifts giving people the vaccine herself. As she plunged needles into arms, she allowed herself to picture "the end of this being the first thing we think about every day. The end of this defining our interactions with humans."

NO END IN SIGHT

As I'm writing this now, in the fall of 2021, it's devastating to say, the end Dara imagined is not yet here.

We don't yet have a vaccine-resistant coronavirus, but it turned out we had enough vaccine-resistant Americans to allow a new, more contagious variant to rampage through the country. Many more Americans died of COVID in 2021 than in 2020.

Several factors combined to make parents feel more anxious, angry, exhausted, and forgotten than ever in the Delta wave. Restrictions like masks lifted in many places before the vaccine was available for children under twelve. Older people, who had been most vulnerable to COVID, were now more likely to be vaccinated. So the age skew of cases changed.

Emergency rooms and pediatric ICUs started filling up with children. Media coverage left some parents with the impression that the Delta variant was more dangerous or deadly to the children who caught it.

In fact, Delta was more contagious but not more serious for young people. Case counts grew. But death, hospitalization, and serious complications, such as debilitating long COVID and multisystem inflammatory disorder, remained vanishingly rare in children. That rarity was actually one of the reasons the approval of the vaccine for children was delayed. Severe complications from COVID were so rare in children under twelve that it required more test subjects and more follow-up time to balance the efficacy with the small risks of the vaccine itself.

Rare doesn't mean nonexistent. More than four million US children tested positive for COVID from March 2020 through the summer of 2021. Around four hundred died.

A THIRD DISRUPTED SCHOOL YEAR

And just like that, a shadow fell over the third school year in a row. Rather than rest, reflect, and recover, districts were once again playing catch-up, in an environment more fraught than ever.

At least by the fall of 2021, compared to the previous year, there was more of a consensus here in the United States that children needed to be in school in person. In this, we had caught up to European and other peer countries. The CDC relaxed recommendations on social distancing so that children everywhere would be able to return five days a week.

We had a new administration that acknowledged science, but there was still zero evident public will or leadership here to prioritize children.

Nowhere did the United States close other businesses and gathering places to keep spread in check so that schools could operate more safely. No one made sure public schools had enough tests to stay open continuously while limiting spread, the way some private schools, private businesses, sports teams, and movie productions were able to do.

And there were growing factions of Americans who opposed vaccines, masks, and tests as a matter of ideology. Republicans in states including Florida, Texas, South Carolina, and Arkansas took steps to ban masking in schools.

In Amador County, in rural Northern California, on the first day of school, a father who opposed masks flew into a rage and hit a teacher multiple times in the face. School board meetings were disrupted by angry mobs of anti-maskers, anti-vaxxers, and those opposed to schools teaching about racism and LGBTQ rights.

With undisclosed political donors backing them, right-wing protesters organized online, made up "watch lists" of school board members, and traveled from outlying counties to come to meetings and yell at board members.

Individual board members, who are often volunteers, got hate mail and death threats. "I was called a demon spawn," Karen Watkins, a first-time school board member in Gwinnett County, Georgia, told me for NPR. "I'm trying to kill our kids by putting on a mask." She was followed to the parking lot after a board meeting and filmed, strange cars were seen in her neighborhood, and a man told her on the phone, "We're coming after you." In late September, the National School Boards Association appealed to President Biden to ask federal law enforcement to intervene in what it considered "acts of domestic terrorism."

Teacher unions came out gingerly in favor of vaccine mandates for educators. But in places where anti-vax sentiment was high, districts feared they wouldn't have the staff needed to stay open if they forced all their food service workers, classroom aides, bus drivers, and maintenance workers to get the shots. They were already experiencing staff shortages because of general post-pandemic labor market upheaval. Massachusetts called out the National Guard to drive school buses.

Rising cases, which again fell unequally on communities of color, combined with the politicization of the pandemic, made Black, Latinx, and Asian American families especially concerned about returning to school in person. And the Delta surge made it more difficult for districts to press those parents to overcome what was being called "school hesitancy." For the fall of 2021, all of the nation's one hundred largest school districts planned to open classes full-time in person, but as Delta surged, most changed their tune to offer remote options as well.

High transmission meant quarantines. Quarantines meant students missing many days of school—because of a lack of testing and because of weak CDC messaging, for months, on the use of testing to limit quarantines. When enough staff members got sick, thousands of schools had to close for a week or so at a time. Early indicators as of the fall of 2021 were that public school enrollment would trend down for the second year in a row, especially in big cities. Some students were going to private and charter schools or suburban districts or homeschooling; others were dropping out for good.

A DELICATE PROCESS OF REPAIR

Ruby summed up her experience of 2020 this way: "I can get through this year, but I can't do this again next year."

As I write this, COVID vaccines for children aged five to eleven have arrived. It's a huge relief. Yet if and when COVID one day calms down to endemic status, it still feels like the curtain has parted on an era of instability.

A paper published in 2006 gives a hint of how long COVID's impacts could linger. Using census data, it traced the fates of Americans who were in utero during the 1918 flu pandemic a century ago. With the caveat that the flu, unlike COVID, took special aim at women of childbearing age, the study found that the children gestated during those nine months grew up to get less schooling and earn less money. The differences were sharper in hotspots, where infection rates were higher. The likelihood of being poor rose as much as 15 percent. Disability rates were 20 percent higher at age sixty-one.

With that in mind, looking ahead, I want to close with two points.

The first is how to redress the wrongs done to children during this time and craft a truly child-centric society.

The second is how to hold in balance the two ideas that this pandemic was a disaster for children and that our children are not damaged goods. We must have hope and talk to children about what happened in a way that expresses our conviction in a better future for them.

To put things right we need to put children at the center of our decision making in a way we never have before in this country.

Attorney Warren Binford is a fearless advocate for children, including migrants detained at the border and survivors of sexual abuse. "Ultimately for me, it's all about kids and the fact that they don't have the political power that you and I have as adults in our society," she tells me.

The UN Convention on the Rights of the Child was adopted in 1989. Since then, national constitutions around the world have increasingly recognized children's rights. This includes both their universal human rights and the special consideration and protection they deserve by virtue of their youth. Children's rights comprise the right to citizenship, the right to health care and education, the right to be raised by their own families if at all possible, and sometimes the right to self-expression and to have their interests heard and represented as well as possible in matters concerning them.

Binford has studied this major legal and philosophical evolution. She calls South Africa's constitution, which came into effect in 1997, exemplary for its detailed and explicit recognition of children's rights. The United States, whose constitution has not been substantively amended for decades, is, no surprise, an outlier here. We are also the only member nation not to have ratified the UN declaration.

What children went through during the pandemic in the United States, I think, is best understood and addressed as a violation of their rights.

And beginning to honor children's rights could transform society for the better in all kinds of ways:

> An expanded vision of civic representation that includes the rights of the nonvoter—perhaps the migrant and refugee as well as the child.
>
> An expanded vision of productivity that values nonmarket contributions—perhaps those of the natural world as well as those of caregivers.
>
> And an expanded vision of public responsibility that requires weighing the long-term future consequences of our actions—one that could transform how we think about the use of resources like fossil fuels or farmland.

Emphasizing and enforcing children's rights might mean overhauling the special education system. Instead of a fight to get kids tested, labeled, and served, what if all schools were required to create individualized education plans by default for all children?

It would for sure mean changing the funding, incentive structure, and tactics of child welfare. If children had the affirmative right to stay with kin, welfare agencies might have to provide families with needed services like housing, income, or drug or mental health counseling. In the current system it's the families of origin who have the burden of proof and of jumping through hoops to regain their children.

This nation could mend the fault lines exposed by this pandemic with a mixture of public and private efforts. The process reminds me of the Japanese art of *kintsugi*, where cracks in pottery are filled in with lacquer mixed with gold.

POST-COVID GROWTH

K. Tsianina Lomawaima writes about American Indian boarding schools, another American phenomenon involving children that was both a social catastrophe and a massive injustice.

Lomawaima tells me that whenever she gave a public talk, she was faced with diametrically opposed reactions. "There'd be at least one Native person who stood up and said, how dare you? They'd be in tears. 'How dare you say anything good about these schools?' The same audience, another Native person in tears: 'How dare you say anything bad about these schools?'"

Without changing her judgment of the schools, she honors the complexity of people's experiences. "Some people did not survive. Others did. And actually, you might even say, came out stronger in the end than before, although that's a tough way to get stronger," she tells me.

What happens to people in a lifetime—especially in the larger cultural or social context—doesn't necessarily get summed up in a way that exactly maps with that spectrum of human experiences. We'll see how this goes as time goes along. But I can see that happening with this pandemic.

Between damned if you do and damned if you don't is this incredible array of actual human beings with actual voices to whom you want to do some justice.

Speaking of coming out stronger, Richard G. Tedeschi, a professor of psychology emeritus at the University of North Carolina at Charlotte, has done some of the key work on what's called posttraumatic growth.

Posttraumatic growth is different from resilience. Resilience is like grass springing up after a footfall—returning to baseline.

Posttraumatic growth is rarer, not automatic. It's like certain tree species with seeds that are released only by the heat of a wildfire.

Posttraumatic growth happens across several dimensions: individually, as people recognize their own strengths that allowed them to survive; socially, when they express gratitude and feel closer to the people who supported them; intellectually and spiritually, as they gain a new perspective on life and clearer priorities.

Based on his clinical practice, Tedeschi suggests this kind of growth can be fostered in others. Parents and caregivers can become "expert companions" to our children as they find their way past the pandemic. This reminds me of what Joseph Kelly, the bereavement counselor, calls "companioning" in the words of Alan Wolfelt, as a way to approach being with people through loss. We can guide the children we love into growth through, and past, this disaster and the disasters to come.

There are five paths to fostering posttraumatic growth, Tedeschi writes: "education, emotional regulation, disclosure, narrative development, and service."

Emotional regulation is a basic toolbox to deal with emotions like sadness, rage, and anxiety without being overwhelmed or stuffing them away. Like the chart on Jonah's refrigerator that suggests he cuddle Teddy the cat or spread out like a star on his bed when he starts to roil inside.

Acts of service can mean helping those less fortunate. Like when Dara and her family choose a different charity to support for each night of Hanukkah. Like when Heather spent part of her own relief check on food for people living in tents and took her son with her to help.

Education, disclosure, and narrative development are different parts of a process that boils down to telling stories: what happened, how we felt about it, what it meant, and what comes next.

I am regularly asking my daughters what they remember about each phase of the pandemic. I don't shy away from talking about the hard parts.

I tell them how proud I am of the positive qualities that the difficulties brought out in them: bravery, flexibility, humor, self-sufficiency, caring.

And because of, not despite, everything they have experienced and witnessed at their young age, I'm helping them imagine a future that turns out better than we could hope.

ACKNOWLEDGMENTS

This book exists because of the foresight and unwavering support of my editor, Benjamin Adams. The task of reporting and writing it kept me somewhat sane during 2020 and 2021, so I count this as a personal favor, not just a professional opportunity. It's been an honor to work with him, Jaime Leifer, Lindsay Fradkoff, Melissa Veronesi, and the team at PublicAffairs a third time.

Thank you to the families, for telling me about some of their toughest days, sometimes on their toughest days.

Thank you to the scholars and other experts who took time away from their work and personal responsibilities to share their expertise with me in the middle of a pandemic.

Crucial encouragement and insight came from Gabe Freiman, Erica Green, Gia Kagan-Trenchard, Alec MacGillis, Brandie Melendez, Linda Rosenbury, Arielle Zibrak, Lydia Denworth, Reem Kassis, Christine Kenneally, Lauren Sandler, all the Invisibles, and the women's circle.

And as always, from my parents, Rodger Kamenetz and Moira Crone.

Thanks to Steve Drummond, my boss, and all my colleagues at National Public Radio. I've learned so much from you. You inspire me.

Thanks to my amazing publicist, Nicole Dewey. And to my assistants, Jill Copeland and Janelle Zagala.

This book could not exist without my children's other caregivers: Emily Kaplan, Heather Dunlop, Zayne Sibley. The staff at Carrig Montessori, Brooklyn Apple, Eden Village Camp, PS 132, PS 110, and GPLESM. And their grandparents, who love them so well.

Thanks to my girls, Lulu and Elvy: they try hard, they find the joy in every day, they are brave and loving.

Adam, жизнь прожить—не поле перейти, but we're crossing it together.

NOTES

The endnotes for this book can be found at anyakamenetz.net.

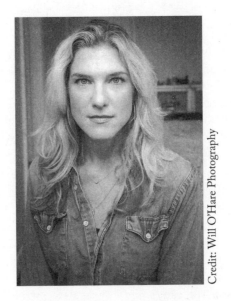

Anya Kamenetz is an education correspondent for NPR. She's contributed to the *New York Times*, the *Washington Post*, *New York Magazine*, and many other publications, and has won multiple awards for her reporting. She is the author of four previous books: *Generation Debt*, *DIY U*, *The Test*, and *The Art of Screen Time*. She lives in Brooklyn with her family.